EAT

TO BEAT

DISEASE

COOKBOOK

**Discover Ultimate Foods &
Recipes That Fights
Chronic Diseases like,
Cancer, Obesity, Diabetes,
Alzheimer, Reduce Aging
& Increase Your Lifespan**

Jason Low

INTRODUCTION

There are dietitian's desire foods, the elite, nutritious and tasty. They are foods that fight diseases that should be in everyone's kitchen simply because they contain wealth of disease fighting substances.

Therefore, put these easily available disease battling foods on the grocery store list today. And ideally, these types of nutritious nibbles ought to replace other, much less healthful, foods, assisting you to overcome diseases while improving the nutrition in your diet.

In life how long we enjoy it—
are out of our own control.
But study, shows that people
in their 90s and beyond, that
eat healthy live even more
longer.

I've compiled the most
compelling and surprising
tips here on how you can eat
to beat disease even in this
epidemic time!

Table of Contents

7-DAY CANCER-FIGHTING MEAL PLAN

Day 1

Breakfast:

BLUEBERRY-ORANGE SMOOTHIE, ENGLISH MUFFIN WITH PEANUT BUTTER:

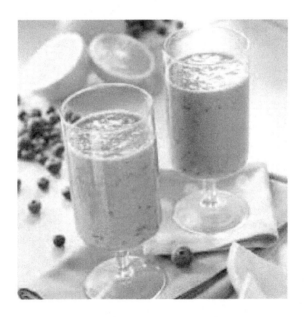

- In a blender

- puree 1/2 cup each orange segments
- frozen blueberries and vanilla
- almond milk with 1/2 frozen banana
- Serve with 1 toasted whole-wheat English muffin spread
- 1 tablespoon peanut butter.

Lunch:

TOMATO SOUP & WHITE BEAN SALAD:

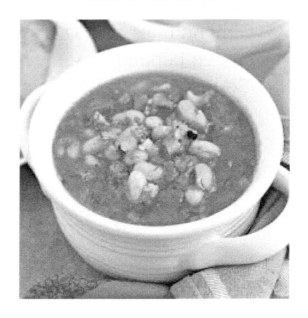

- In a bowl
- toss 3/4 cup rinsed drained white beans
- 1 tbsp each diced red onion

- chopped basil and chopped parsley
- Dress with 1 tbsp low-fat balsamic vinaigrette
- Serve with 1 1/2 cups tomato soup (such as Muir Glen Tomato-Basil)
- Whole-grain roll.

Dinner:

SPINACH PIZZA WITH ROMAINE SALAD:

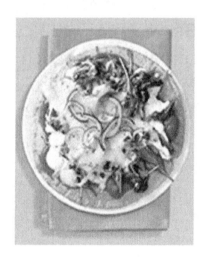

- Thaw 5 ounces frozen spinach; squeeze and chop.
- Over medium heat, sautée;
- 1 crushed garlic clove in 2 teaspoons olive oil for 30 seconds.

- Add spinach and a pinch of salt; sautée; 2 minutes.
- Spread 2 tbsp tomato paste (save rest for tacos, day 2, and Bolognese, day 3) on an 8-inch whole-wheat pita; toast 2 minutes.
- Combine spinach with 5 tbsp part-skim ricotta and black pepper; spread over pizza
- top with 2 tbsp grated part-skim mozzarella.
- Top with 1 tbsp diced red onion; broil 3 minutes.
- Serve with salad of romaine, chickpeas, cherry tomatoes,

shredded carrots and 1 1/2 tbsp low-fat Italian vinaigrette.

Day 2:

Breakfast:

SCRAMBLED EGGS WITH BROCCOLI:

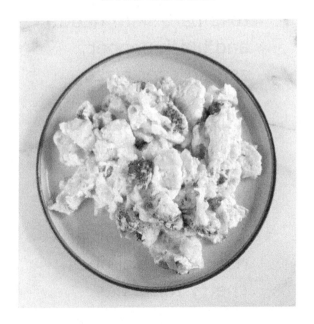

- Beat 2 eggs with 1 tsp water
- 1 tsp grated Parmesan, salt and pepper. In a pan
- Heat 2 tsp olive oil. Sautée
- 1/4 cup sliced onion
- 1/4 tsp dried thyme for 3 minutes
- Add 1/2 cup chopped broccoli; sautée; 2 minutes
- Add eggs
- scramble until set
- Serve with 1 slice whole-wheat toast and 8 oz OJ.

Lunch:

PASTA SALAD WITH SALMON:

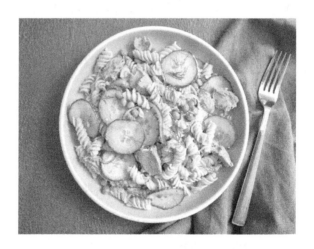

- Cook 2 oz whole-wheat pasta as directed on package. In a bowl
- whisk 1 tbsp chopped kalamata olives
- 2 tsp each olive oil and lemon juice
- 1 tsp Dijon mustard

- Add 1/4 cup each canned pink salmon, chickpeas and halved cherry tomatoes
- Toss in cooked pasta and
- 1 cup baby arugula.
- Serve with lemon wedge.

Dinner:

CHICKEN TACOS WITH MANGO & JICAMA:

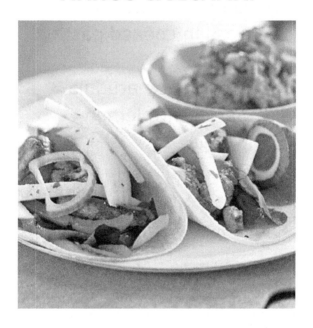

- In a skillet, warm 1/2 tsp olive oil over medium heat
- Stir in 1 chopped, cooked chicken breast

- 1 tsp each tomato paste (reserve remainder for Bolognese, day 3) and tomato sauce
- 1/2 tsp chili powder. Sautée; 2 minutes
- Add 1 tbsp each chopped onion and fresh cilantro
- 1 tsp lime juice and a pinch of salt
- Top each of 2 warm corn tortillas with 2 tbsp warm low-fat refried beans
- half of chicken mixture
- 2 tbsp shredded romaine
- 1 tbsp salsa
- 2 tsp low-fat sour cream

- Serve with salad of 1/2 cup each sliced mango
- Jicama sticks sprinkled with 2 tsp lime juice and 1/2 tsp chili powder.

Day 3

Breakfast:

CEREAL BAR, PEAR & LATTE:

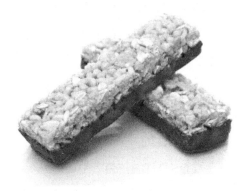

- Have 1 all-natural fruit-and-nut bar (get one with at least 3 grams fiber and 4 g protein)
- 1 medium pear
- 1 small skim latte.

Lunch:

AVOCADO, SPINACH & SWISS SANDWICH:

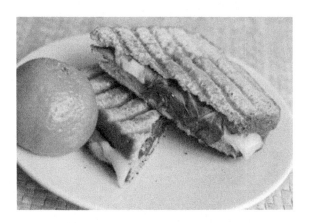

- Mash 1/2 avocado

- 1/2 tsp lemon juice
- a pinch of black pepper
- Spread on 1 slice whole-wheat toast
- Top with 1/2 cup baby spinach
- 1/4 cup thinly sliced bell pepper
- 2 slices low-fat Swiss and 1 more slice toast
- Serve with 1 cup red grapes.

Dinner:

TURKEY BOLOGNESE WITH TRICOLOR SALAD:

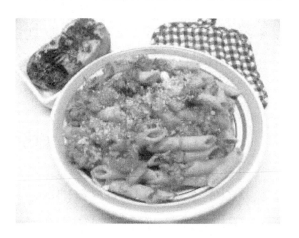

- Brown 16 oz lean ground turkey in 2 tsp olive oil over high heat. In a food processor
- 2 celery stalks
- 1 carrot
- 1 red onion
- 2 garlic cloves; transfer to pan

- Add 2 tsp oil
- A pinch of salt. Cook, covered, over medium-low heat for 8 minutes
- Add turkey, 1 cup each tomato sauce and chicken stock
- 1 tbsp tomato paste; simmer, partly covered, 10 minutes
- Add 3 tbsp 1 percent milk; simmer 5 minutes
- Mix 1 1/2 cups cooked whole-wheat spaghetti with 1 cup sauce
- Top with 1 tsp Parmesan. In a bowl
- mix 1/2 cup each romaine, arugula, radicchio and sliced cucumbers

- Drizzle with 1 tbsp low-fat vinaigrette.

Day 4

Breakfast:

ALMOND BUTTER & BANANA TOAST:

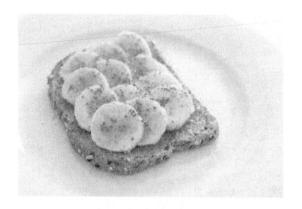

- Spread 1 tbsp almond butter on 1 slice whole-wheat toast

- Top with 1/2 sliced banana
- Serve with 8 oz skim green-tea latte.

Lunch:

WALDORF CHICKEN SALAD:

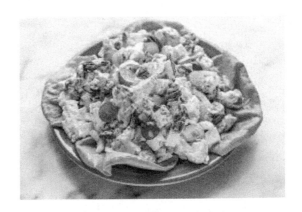

- In a bowl, whisk 1/4 cup low-fat plain yogurt
- 1/2 tbsp mayo, 1 tsp lemon juice

- 1/2 tsp mustard
- a pinch each of salt and pepper
- Add 3/4 cup chopped chicken breast
- 1/4 cup each chopped apples
- red grapes and celery
- 2 tsp diced onion
- Serve over 1 1/2 cups romaine
- 1 tbsp chopped almonds
- A whole-grain roll on the side.

Dinner:

MINESTRONE WITH SQUASH, BEANS & KALE:

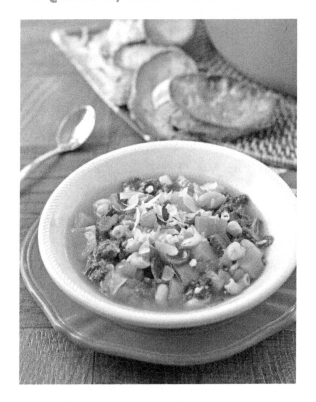

- Dice 1 onion
- 1 carrot
- 1 celery stalk

- 1 garlic clove. In a pan, sautee
- vegetables in 2 tbsp olive oil for 5 minutes
- add 1 quart low-sodium chicken broth
- 2 cups water
- one 15-oz can chopped plum tomatoes with juice
- 1/2 tsp salt; bring to a boil
- Add 3 cups chopped kale
- 2 cups cubed butternut squash
- 1 1/2 cups each whole-wheat elbow macaroni, chopped zucchini and kidney beans; simmer

until tender, 15 to 20 minutes

- Add 1/4 cup pesto
- 2 tbsp chopped fresh parsley
- black pepper to taste
- Serve 2 cups soup
- 1 tbsp grated Parmesan
- 1 whole-grain breadstick. (You can freeze soup for up to 1 month.)

Day 5

Breakfast:

CEREAL WITH RAISINS & ALMONDS; HALF GRAPEFRUIT WITH HONEY:

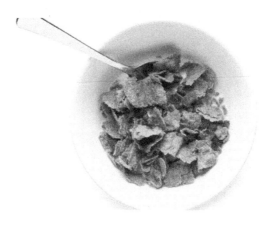

- Mix 1 cup whole-grain cereal
- 1/2 cup 1 percent milk
- 2 tbsp each raisins and sliced almonds

- Serve with 1/2 grapefruit drizzled
- 2 tsp honey.

Lunch:

ZIPPY EGG-SALAD SANDWICH:

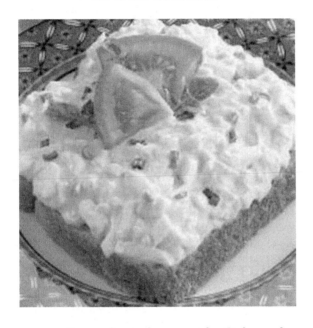

- In a bowl, mash 2 hard-boiled eggs
- 1 hard-boiled egg white
- 2 tsp each hummus and mayonnaise

- 1/2 tsp each Dijon mustard and lemon juice
- 1/4 tsp turmeric. Spoon between
- 2 slices whole-grain toast with
- 1/4 cup baby spinach and
- 1/2 sliced tomato
- Serve with
- 1/2 cup carrot sticks and
- 1 orange.

Dinner:

STEAK SALAD:

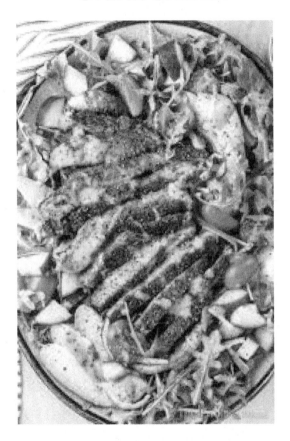

- In a skillet over high heat

- sear 4 oz flank steak in
- 1/2 tsp vegetable oil until medium-rare, 3 to 4 minutes per side
- In a bowl, whisk 1 diced scallion with
- 2 tsp olive oil
- 2 tsp red wine vinegar
- 1 tsp Dijon mustard
- 1/4 tsp each salt and pepper
- Set aside 1 tsp dressing
- Add 1 1/2 cups torn romaine to bowl with dressing, then
- add 1/2 cup each halved grape tomatoes and chopped bell pepper, and
- 1/3 cup corn; toss
- Top with sliced steak

- 1/4 chopped avocado and reserved 1 tsp dressing
- Brush 1 slice whole-grain toast with
- 1/2 tsp olive oil and
- 1 tbsp grated Parmesan; broil until melted, 1 to 2 minutes and Serve.

Day 6

Breakfast:

BERRY-COCONUT OATMEAL:

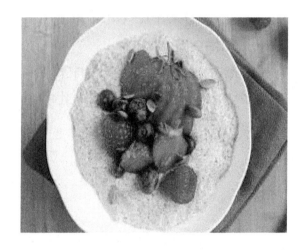

- In a pan, simmer
- 1/2 cup rolled oats
- 1 tbsp oat bran and
- 1/4 tsp cinnamon with
- 1 cup 1 percent milk
- 1/2 cup water and

- a pinch of salt for 6 minutes
- In a skillet, toast 3 tbsp shredded unsweetened coconut with
- 1 tbsp brown sugar over medium heat until sugar melts, 1 minute
- Top oatmeal with coconut and
- 1/8 cup fresh raspberries.

Lunch:

TOFU SALAD:

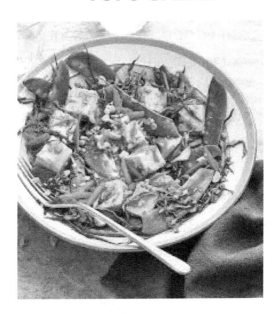

- Toss 4 oz cubed firm tofu
- 1/2 cup each steamed broccoli and sugar snap peas
- 1/4 cup halved grape tomatoes

- 2 tbsp sesame-ginger dressing
- Sprinkle with 1/2 tsp toasted sesame seeds and
- 1 diced scallion
- Serve with 3/4 cup cooked brown rice drizzled with
- 1 tsp reduced-sodium soy sauce and
- 1/2 tsp sesame oil.

Dinner:

TOMATO-PESTO TILAPIA WITH GARLICKY KALE:

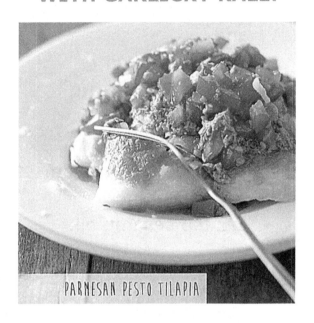

PARMESAN PESTO TILAPIA

- Microwave 1 medium red potato until tender, 10 minutes
- Place a 6-oz fillet of tilapia (or other flaky

white fish) in a baking pan
- Mix 1/2 tbsp each pesto and chopped fresh parsley
- spread over fish; drizzle with
- 1/2 tsp olive oil and season with
- a pinch of black pepper
- Top with 1/2 cup halved grape tomatoes
- Broil until fish is tender, 6 to 8 minutes.
- In a pan, sautée; 1 tsp olive oil with
- 1 crushed garlic clove over medium heat
- Add 2 cups kale and
- a pinch of salt; sauée; until wilted

- Add 1 tbsp chicken stock or water; cook, covered, until tender, 2 to 3 minutes
- Slice potato into rounds;
- Top with fish, tomatoes and kale.

Day 7

Breakfast:

PEAR PANCAKES WITH HONEY:

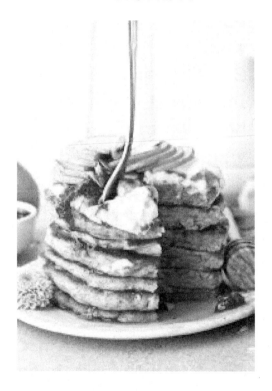

- Whisk 1/2 cup whole-wheat pastry flour with

- 2 tbsp all-purpose flour
- 1/2 tsp baking soda
- a pinch each of salt and cinnamon
- Mix in 1/2 cup low-fat buttermilk and 1 beaten egg
- Slice 1 pear.
- In a skillet over medium heat, warm 1 tsp vegetable oil
- drop 1/4 cup batter into pan
- top with 2 slices pear
- Cook 1 to 2 minutes per side.
- Top 4 cakes with
- 1/4 cup nonfat plain Greek yogurt, remaining pear slices and
- 2 tsp honey mixed with

- 1/2 tsp lemon juice. (Freeze extras.)

Lunch:

TABBOULEH, HUMMUS & PITA:

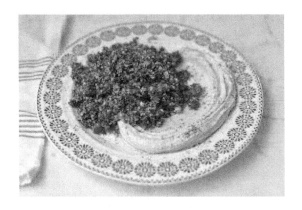

- Cook 1/4 cup fine bulgur wheat as directed on package with
- A pinch each of salt, ground cumin and dried mint. Cover

- Remove from heat. Let sit 25 minutes
- Stir in 1/4 cup each diced fresh parsley and tomato
- 1 diced scallion
- 1 tbsp lemon juice and
- 2 tsp olive oil
- Serve with 1/2 whole-wheat pita
- 1/4 cup hummus and 1 apple.

Dinner:

CHICKEN KEBABS WITH COUSCOUS:

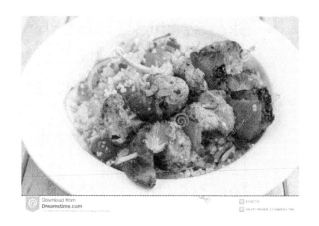

- Whisk 1/2 cup low-fat plain yogurt with
- 1 tsp lemon juice
- 1/2 tsp each olive oil and curry powder
- 1 crushed garlic clove and
- 1/4 tsp each turmeric and salt

- Stir in 4 oz cubed chicken breast; cover and refrigerate 2 to 12 hours.
- Skewer chicken. Brush with 1 tsp olive oil
- broil on rack, turning occasionally, until cooked through, about 15 minutes
- Top 3/4 cup cooked whole-wheat couscous with chicken, and drizzle with 2 tbsp low-fat plain yogurt
- Serve with salad of 1/4 cup each sliced cucumber, bell pepper, plum tomato and chopped fresh parsley

- And 1 tbsp diced red onion.
- For dressing, whisk a pinch each of salt, pepper and sugar with
- 1 tsp each olive oil and red wine vinegar.

When You Wake Up:

Turmeric Latte

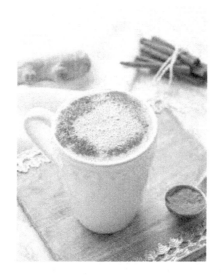

- Grate 3/4-inch fresh peeled ginger root and 1/2-inch turmeric root into a mortar.

- Add one teaspoon coconut oil to create a paste. In saucepan, simmer paste with 1/2 cup full-fat coconut milk, 1/2 cup coconut water, 1/2 teaspoon cloves for four minutes. Strain and enjoy.

Pre-Breakfast:

Green Juice

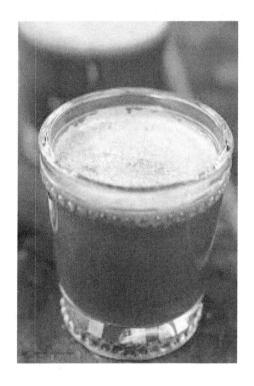

Juice one-inch each fresh

turmeric and ginger, one

handful each spinach and

kale, one cucumber, one cup

filtered water. Drink half,

and save the other half.

Breakfast: Energy

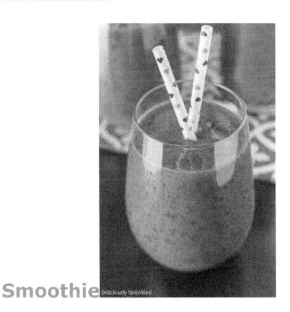

Smoothie

- Blend 1/2 cup soaked almonds

- 1/4 cup soaked cashews, 1/2 avocado

- 1/2 cucumber, two handfuls of spinach, one handful of kale

- Three tablespoons coconut oil

- One tablespoon each sunflower and chia seeds

- One cup almond milk.

- Drink half, and save the other half.

Mid-Morning:Juice

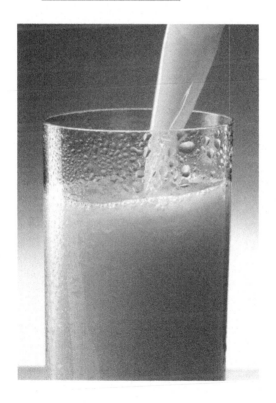

Enjoy the second glass of

your green juice.

Gut-Healing Soup

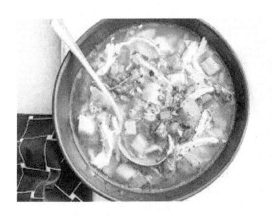

- Cook one cup lentils.

  Sauté four cloves garlic

- One chopped onion

- One diced sweet potato

- Two diced carrots.

- Add one cup broth and
  cook until al dente.

- Blend lentils, broth, one
  avocado

- One handful spinach,
  one bell pepper, and
  one handful cashews
  until smooth.

- Makes two servings.

Mid-afternoon:

Smoothie

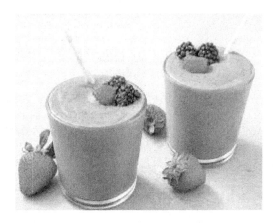

Enjoy the second glass of

your energy smoothie.

Dinner:

Warming Squash Soup

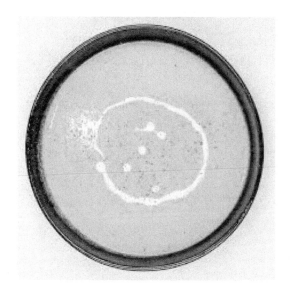

Simmer one peeled and

chopped butternut squash in

1 1/4 cup organic, low-

sodium veggie broth. Add

one diced onion and 12

ounces' coconut milk.

Simmer until squash is soft,

then blend. Add salt, pepper,

and nutmeg to taste. _Makes_

two servings.

Raisins:

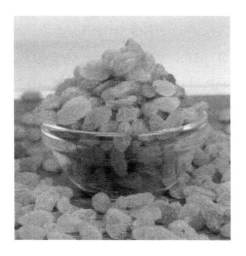

Raisins are a tasty natural snack that can be eaten on their own or added to a variety of recipes, such as oatmeal raisin cookies. In addition to being so versatile, they're also simple to make.

Serving Suggestion: Suggested storage containers for air-dried raisins include Mylar bags, Tupperware, and glass canning jars with an oxygen absorber. Homemade Raisins made this way and saved in an airtight container can be saved in a cool, dry place for several months.

Ingredients:

- 500 gams green grapes
- 3-4 water for boiling.

Directions:

- Collect all the required ingredients.
- Take green grapes and remove the larger

stems from your grapes.

- Rinse the grapes under running water to wash them.
- Wash thoroughly for 3-4 times.
- Take enough water in a deep pan for blanching.
- Before drying your grapes, you'll want to blanch them. You can skip this step if you want, but blanching your grapes first softens the skins and helps them dry evenly. And it only takes a minute. Do not boil the water is just heat it.

- When the water starts heating, drop the grapes.
- After 2-3 minutes, the grapes will starts floating above the water.
- When the grapes will boil over and the crack has come in them too. Switch off the flame.
- Do not over boil the grapes.
- As soon as the grapefruit starts floating and all our grape exploded from the center, take them out from the water.

- Take out the grapes from water using sieve or spoon.
- Let them cool for 5-7 minutes.
- Take a plate/tray or basket and spread cheesecloth/kitchen towel/cotton cloth.
- Spread the grapes over the cloth.
- Place the tray outside in a dry sunny place. Take the tray inside in the night if it is foggy. Every day keep it out in the morning and take it inside in the night. Keep rotating the fruit for even exposure to the sun. It takes around 1

to 2 days depending on the strength of the sun rays.

- Once the grapes have dried to the point of becoming raisins, take the tray inside and place the raisins in an airtight container. Store the container in a cool place or refrigerate.

Notes:

- Over-ripe grapes will take longer to dry and may rot before drying. It's preferable to have slightly under-ripe, yet sweet, grapes.

- Watch for dampness or rot. If a few grapes go bad, remove them immediately from the tray and spread close by fruit out to dry. Remember that drying grapes will shrivel up and get small, not turn to mush and rot.
- Professionals often create raisins by dangling bunches of fruit from the string or even wire and enabling them to dried out. This is tougher than employing a toned tray but functions better because the fresh fruit

has maximum
atmosphere exposure.

BLACK CURRENTS:

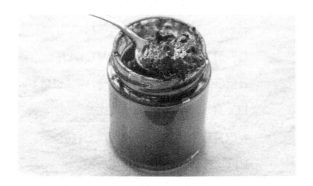

This easy recipe uses the
whole fruit for a tart, rich
preserve that sets well. It's
excellent on crisp toasted rye
bread, or spooned with
yoghurt onto porridge in the
morning. You'll need a sugar
thermometer for this recipe.

Ingredients:

- 300g/10½oz fresh blackcurrants
- 300g/10½oz granulated or caster sugar
- 1 small lemon, juice only.

Directions:

- Pick all the stalks from the blackcurrants, place the fruit in a saucepan, cover with 250ml/9fl oz. water and bring to the boil. Simmer for 20 minutes, or until the skins of the currants are very tender and the liquid has almost evaporated.

- Add the sugar and lemon juice, bring to the boil then cook until the mixture reaches 105C/220F on a sugar thermometer.
- Leave to cool for a few minutes then pour into hot, clean jars and seal immediately.

Do you want to go alkaline? Good for you, I've been practicing this lifestyle for years and have created some pretty tasty recipes, if I may say so myself. Going alkaline doesn't mean cutting foods completely out of your diet, so let's not focus on elimination. Rather, think of all the delicious, fresh and healthy foods you can eat to promote alkalinity. To help you through it, I've compiled a seven-day meal plan with my favorite alkaline recipes (using ingredients you already probably work with all the time) to help get you started. Prepare to feel more energized and pain-free in no time!

DAY ONE

Breakfast: **Strawberry Coco Chia Quinoa**

Breakfast

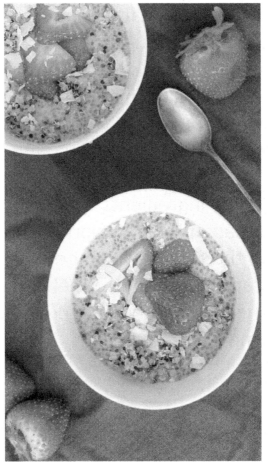

Ingredients:

- 1 cup cooked quinoa

- 5 tbsp. chia seeds
- 1 ½ cup almond, coconut or hemp milk
- ½ cup quartered strawberries + 4 sliced strawberries
- 2 pitted date
- 2 tbsp. almond pieces
- 2 tbsp. unsweetened shredded coconut flakes.

Directions:

The night time before, cook quinoa and prepare blood chia by merging the strawberries, cashew milk, and two dates in the blender and blending until smooth. Put the mixture in to a jar plus add chia seed products. Mix well till all chia seed products are covered along with the liquid. Protect with lid plus refrigerate overnight. Each morning, place chia seed products in bowl, include the quinoa plus strawberry slices, walnuts, and shredded coconut and enjoy!

Lunch:

Sweet and Savory Salad

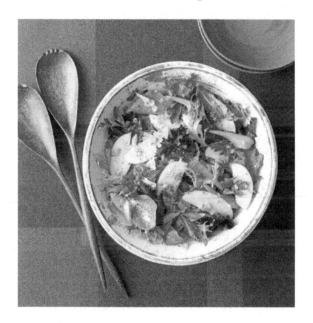

Ingredients:

- 1 large head of butter lettuce
- ½ cucumber, sliced
- 1 pomegranate, seeded or 1/3 cup seeds
- 1 avocado, cubed

- ¼ cup shelled pistachios, chopped.

Dressing Ingredients:

- ¼ cup apple cider vinegar
- ½ cup extra virgin olive oil
- 1 garlic clove, minced.

Directions:

Hand tear the butter lettuce into a salad bowl. Add the rest of the ingredients and toss with the salad dressing.

DAY TWO

Non-Dairy Apple Parfait

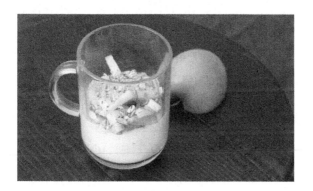

Ingredients:

- ½ cup soaked raw cashews (soak 20 mins- 1 hour)
- ½ cup unsweetened almond or coconut milk
- ½ tsp. vanilla
- 1 cup chopped apple
- 1/3 cup rolled gluten- free oats, uncooked

- 1 tbsp. hemp seeds.

Directions:

Combine cashews, almond milk, and vanilla in a blender and blend until smooth. Layer ingredients in a small cup: heaping spoon of cashew cream, spoonful of apples, top with oats and hemp seeds and enjoy!

Lunch:

Savory Avocado Wrap

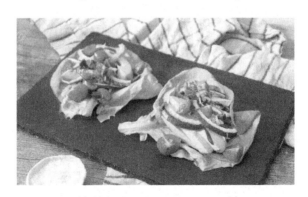

Ingredients:

- 1 butter lettuce or collard leaf bunch
- ½ avocado
- 1 tsp. chopped basil
- Small handful of spinach
- 1 tsp. cilantro, chopped
- ¼ red onion, diced
- 1 tomato, sliced or chopped
- Sea salt & pepper.

Directions:

Spread avocado onto leaf and sprinkle with basil, cilantro, red onion, tomato, salt and pepper and add spinach. Fold in half and enjoy!

DAY THREE

Breakfast:

Almond Butter Crunch Berry Smoothie

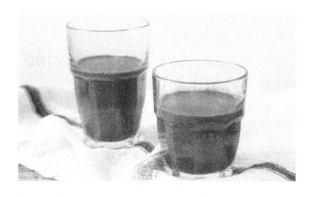

Ingredients:

- 2 cups fresh spinach
- 2 cups almond milk, unsweetened
- 1 cup of any of the following (frozen mixed berries, strawberries or grapes)

- 1 banana (peeled and frozen)
- 4 tbsp. raw almond butter
- 1 tbsp. chia.

Directions:

Blend spinach and almond milk first. Then add remaining ingredients except chia, and blend. Add chia once all is smooth – then blend on a very low speed to mix. If you don't have a variable speed blender, mix chia in with the rest of the ingredients by hand. Let sit for a few minutes for the chia seeds to expand, then enjoy.

Lunch:

Kale Pesto Pasta

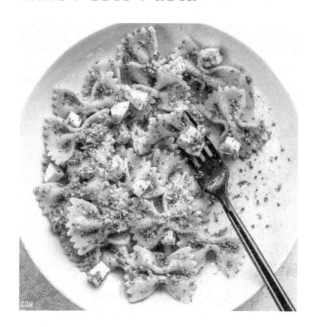

Ingredients:

- 1 bunch kale
- 2 cups fresh basil
- 1/4 cup extra virgin olive oil
- 1/2 cup walnuts
- 2 limes, fresh squeezed

Sea salt and pepper.

- 1 zucchini, noodled (spiralizer)
- Optional: garnish with sliced asparagus, spinach leaves, and tomato.

Directions:

The night before, soak walnuts to improve absorption. Put all ingredients in a blender or food processor, and blend until you get a cream consistency. Add to zucchini noodles and enjoy!

DAY FOUR

Apple and Almond Butter Oats:

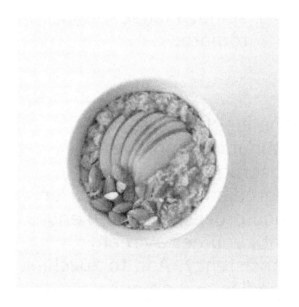

Ingredients:

- 2 cups gluten-free oats
- 1 ½ cups coconut milk

- 1/3 cup raw almond butter
- 1 cup grated green apple
- 1 tsp. cinnamon.

Directions:

Add the oats, coconut milk and almond butter into a bowl and mix well. Stir in the grated apple; cover the bowl with a lid or plastic wrap and place in the refrigerator. Refrigerate overnight. If the oats get too thick, add some coconut milk to them. Garnish with cinnamon powder.

Lunch:

Green Goddess Bowl with Avocado Cumin Dressing:

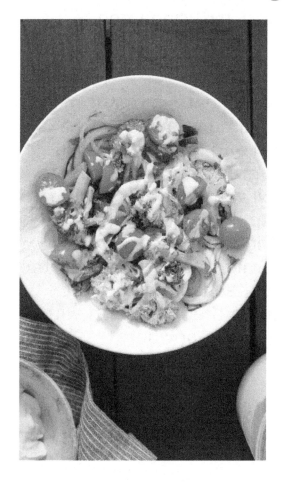

Ingredients:

- 1 avocado
- 1 tbsp. cumin powder
- 2 limes, fresh squeezed
- 1 cup filtered water
- ¼ tsp. sea salt
- 1 tbsp. extra virgin olive oil
- dash cayenne pepper
- Optional: ¼ tsp. smoked paprika.

Ingredients for Tahini Lemon Dressing:

- ¼ cup tahini (sesame butter)
- ½ cup filtered water (more if you desire thinner, less for thicker)
- ½ lemon, fresh squeezed
- 1 clove minced garlic

- ¾ tsp. sea salt (Celtic grey, Himalayan, Redmond Real Salt)
- 1 tbsp. extra virgin olive oil
- Black pepper to taste.

Ingredients for salad:

- 3 cups kale, chopped
- ½ cup broccoli florets, chopped
- ½ zucchini (make noodles with spiralizer)
- ½ cup kelp noodles, soaked and drained
- 1/3 cup cherry tomatoes, halved
- 2 tbsp. hemp seeds.

Directions:

Lightly steam kale and broccoli (flash steam for 4 minutes), set aside. Mix zucchini noodles and kelp noodles and toss with a generous serving of smoked avocado cumin dressing. Add cherry tomatoes and toss again. Plate the steamed kale and broccoli and drizzle them with lemon tahini dressing. Top kale and broccoli with the dressed noodles and tomatoes and sprinkle the whole dish with hemp seeds.

Breakfast:

Berry Good Spinach Power Smoothie

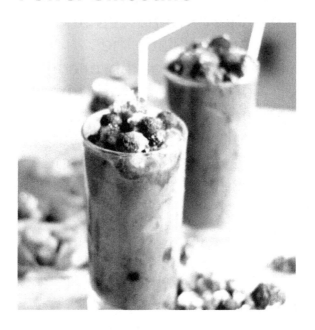

Ingredients:

- 2 cups fresh spinach
- 2 cups unsweetened almond milk
- 1 cup frozen mixed berries

- 1 frozen banana
- 1 tbsp. coconut oil
- ½ tsp. cinnamon
- 2 tbsp. raw almond butter.

Directions:

Blend spinach and almond milk first, then add remaining ingredients and blend.

Lunch:

Quinoa Burrito Bowl:

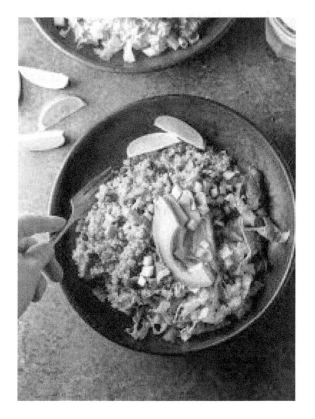

Ingredients:

- 1 cup quinoa (or brown rice)
- 2 15-oz cans of black or adzuki beans
- 4 green onions (scallions), sliced
- 2 limes, fresh juiced
- 4 garlic cloves, minced
- 1 heaping tsp. cumin
- 2 avocados, sliced
- small handful of cilantro, chopped.

Directions:

Cook quinoa or rice. While cooking, warm beans over low heat. Stir in onions, lime juice, garlic and cumin and let flavors combine for 10-15 minutes. When quinoa is done cooking, divide into individual serving bowls. Top

with beans, avocado and
cilantro.

DAY SIX

Quinoa Morning Porridge:

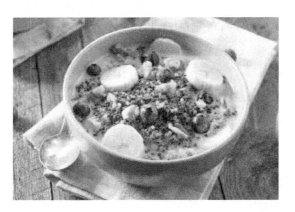

Ingredients:

- ½ cup rinsed quinoa
- 1 15 oz. can of coconut
  milk
- 1 tsp. cinnamon

- 1 tsp. chia seeds
- 1 tsp. hemp seeds.

Directions:

Combine all ingredients except hemp seeds and simmer for 10-15 minutes until liquid is absorbed. Sprinkle with hemp seeds.

<u>Lunch:</u>

Thai Quinoa Salad:

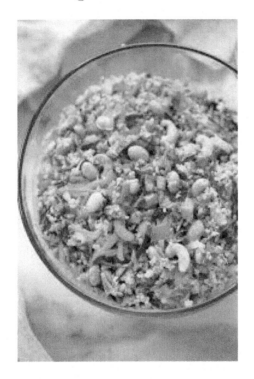

Ingredients for dressing:

- 1 tbsp. sesame seeds
- 1 tsp. chopped garlic

- 1 tsp. lemon, fresh juiced
- 3 tsp. apple cider vinegar
- 2 tsp. tamari, gluten-free
- ¼ cup tahini (sesame butter)
- 1 pitted date
- ½ tsp. salt
- ½ tsp. toasted sesame oil.

Ingredients for salad:

- 1 cup of quinoa, steamed
- 1 large handful of arugula
- 1 tomato, sliced
- ¼ red onion, diced.

Directions:

- In a small blender, add the following: ¼ cup + 2 tbsp.
- Filtered water, then the rest of ingredients. Blend. Steam 1 cup of quinoa in a steamer or rice cooker, then set aside. Combine, quinoa, arugula, sliced tomatoes, diced red onion, onto a serving plate or bowl, add Thai dressing, and hand mix with a spoon and serve.

DAY SEVEN

Breakfast:

Alkaline Warrior Chia Breakfast

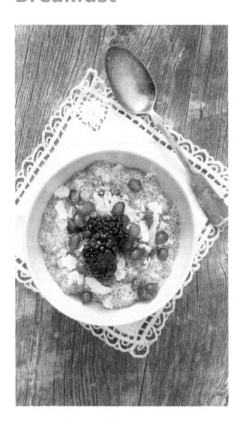

Ingredients:

- 1 cup unsweetened almond or coconut milk
- 4 tbsp. of chia seeds
- ½ tsp. vanilla
- ½ tsp. cinnamon
- 1 tbsp. unsweetened shredded coconut flakes
- ¼ cup chopped nuts (almonds, cashews or hemp seeds).

Directions:

- The night before, combine milk and chia seeds in a mason jar. Add vanilla, cinnamon and chopped nuts. Cover with lid and shake the mixture until it's combined. Refrigerate overnight. The next morning, shake or stir the mixture and divide into 2-3 bowls. Top with optional fresh fruit, coconut shreds or more chopped nuts.

Lunch:

Asian Sesame Dressing and Noodles

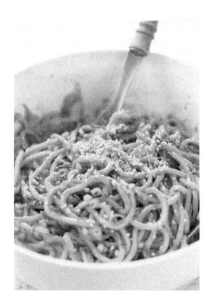

Ingredients for dressing:

- 2 tbsp. tahini (sesame butter)
- 2 tsp. tamari (gluten-free)
- ½ tsp. liquid coconut nectar (Coconut Secrets brand)
- ½ tsp. lemon, fresh squeezed 1 clove garlic, minced.

Ingredients for noodle salad:

- 1 scallion, chopped
- 1 tbsp. raw sesame seeds (topping)
- Optional: sliced red bell pepper and/or carrot.

Directions:

- Choose one of the following for noodles: Kelp Noodles (1 bag) or 1 Zucchini (use spiralizer or vegetable peeler)
- Inside a mixing bowl, blend all the dressing up ingredients and completely mix with a spoon. Make your zucchini noodles with a spiralizer or, if using kelp noodles, place in hot water for ten minutes to wash off the water they are packed with, allowing them to separate and soften. Add the Asian Sesame dressing up to the noodles and scallions,

and mix thoroughly. Include sesame seeds on the top, and serve.

- I really hope you truly enjoy these alkaline quality recipes. Do this for one week, and if you are just like nearly all of my clients, you are heading to feel so great you are not going to actually want to go back! In case you are caring the energy and perhaps, the few extra pounds you might shed!

100-PERCENT HEALTHY MADE EASY

The best thing about the particular alkaline diet is usually that you do not have to depend calories or carbohydrates — it's just about all about nourishment, not really deprivation. "It is not about being vegetarian, but for the reason that alkaline diet is regarding consuming meals that recover your gut, this can make any kind of those diet plans even more efficient. The main element is in order to reset your body along with a seven-day detox before starting the healthy diet. Placing rocket fuel in to a beat-up old vehicle isn't going in order to transform it into the rocket. "You very first have to unclog and rebalance your own systems to restart your body directly into a state exactly where it can operate optimally." Then your stubborn pounds will surely start falling out of your frame.

GOLDEN MILK:

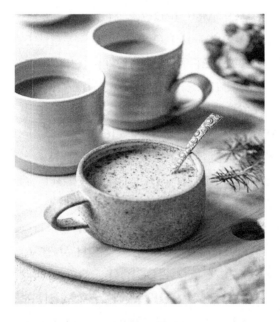

How to Make Golden Milk – 3 Different Ways

Ingredients: 1

Using Ground Turmeric or Turmeric Powder

- 2 ½ cups unsweetened almond milk
- 1 ½ teaspoons ground turmeric powder
- ½ teaspoon ground ginger
- A tablespoon of coconut oil (or ghee)
- A pinch of black pepper
- Maple syrup to taste (optional)

Direction: 1

- Mix everything in a small saucepan and cook until it starts simmering.

Ingredients: 2

Using Fresh Turmeric

- 2 ½ cups unsweetened almond milk or coconut milk
- 2 inches of sliced fresh turmeric root
- 1 inch sliced fresh ginger root
- 1 tablespoon of coconut oil (or ghee)
- A pinch of black pepper
- 1 tablespoon of maple syrup or honey (optional)

Direction: 2

Mix unsweetened homemade almond milk with fresh turmeric root, fresh ginger root, a stick of cinnamon, a pinch of black pepper and a bit coconut oil in saucepan and cook (while I stir constantly) it in medium heat just until it starts simmering.

Turmeric Golden Milk

- 2 ½ cups unsweetened and full fat almond or coconut milk
- 1 stick cinnamon or 1/4 teaspoon ground cinnamon more as garnish at the end
- 2 inches' fresh turmeric sliced or 1 ½ teaspoon ground turmeric spice

- 1-inch fresh ginger sliced or ½ teaspoon ground ginger
- 1 tablespoon coconut oil
- Pinch of black pepper
- 1 tablespoon maple syrup or honey or more to taste

Directions:

- Place milk, cinnamon stick, turmeric, ginger, coconut oil, and black pepper in a small saucepan.

- Cook, stirring frequently, until warm but not boiling.

- Give it a taste and add in your sweetener.

- If you used fresh turmeric and ginger, strain it to your cups. If not, divide it in two mugs.

- If preferred, sprinkle with ground cinnamon. Serve.

BULGUR SALAD WITH HERBS AND CHICKPEAS:

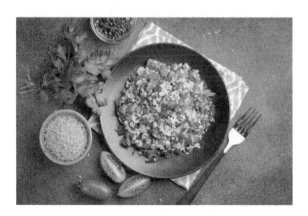

Ingredients:

- 1 cup bulgur
- 1½ cups boiling water
- ¼ cup bottled lemon juice
- ¼ cup olive oil
- ½ tsp. salt
- ½ tsp. ground black pepper
- ½ tsp. ground cinnamon
- ½ tsp. garlic powder
- ½ tsp. ground coriander
- ½ cup flat-leaf parsley, roughly torn by hand
- ¼ cup spearmint leaves, roughly torn by hand
- 2 cups cherry tomatoes, cut in half

- 1 15-oz. can chickpeas, drained and rinsed

Directions:

- Place bulgur in a large heatproof bowl. Carefully pour boiling water over bulgur, and cover bowl with plastic wrap or aluminum foil. Allow the bulgur to steam in bowl for at least 30 minutes.

- Just before the bulgur is done steaming, put lemon juice, olive oil, salt, pepper, cinnamon, garlic powder, and coriander in a jar with a lid. Tightly close lid and

shake jar to combine
ingredients.

- Remove cover on the
  bowl and pour dressing
  over the bulgur. Stir to
  mix dressing with the
  bulgur. Add parsley,
  spearmint, cherry
  tomatoes, and
  chickpeas. Stir to
  combine all ingredients.
  You can eat the bulgur
  salad immediately or
  chill at least 1 hour (or
  overnight) to allow the
  flavors to meld better.

OVERNIGHT MUESLI:

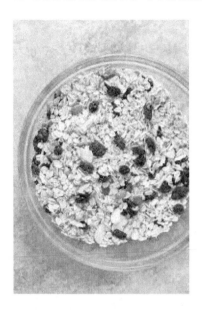

Ingredients:

- 2 cups rolled oats (old fashioned, not instant)
- ¼ cup unsweetened coconut flakes
- ¼ cup raw almonds
- 1/ 2cup chopped dried figs

- 1 granny smith apple (per serving)
- ½ teaspoon ground cinnamon (per serving)
- ¼ cup cow's or almond milk or kefir (per serving, optional)

Directions:

- In a medium glass or ceramic bowl, combine the oats with the next 3 ingredients (through dried figs). Add in 2 cups of water. Mix well and cover with a plate. Let mixture sit at room temperature overnight.

- In the morning, place 1 to 1½ cup of mixture in a bowl, grate the apple

on top of mixture,
sprinkle the cinnamon,
add milk and a little
honey (if using).
Transfer unused mixture
to a tightly sealed
container and
refrigerate. This will
keep in the refrigerator
for 4-5 days.

GINGERED TUNA AND GREENS STIR-FRY:

Ingredients:

- 1 tablespoon canola,
  peanut or grape seed
  oil, divided
- 1 large bunch kale,
  stems removed and

coarsely chopped or
torn
- 1/4teaspoon sea salt
- 2 garlic cloves, thinly
  sliced
- 1 tablespoon freshly
  chopped ginger
- 5 green onions, thinly
  sliced (bulbs and leaves
  separated)
- 1 large red pepper, cut
  into thin slices
- 1-pound fresh tuna
  steak, cut into bit size
  pieces
- ½ tablespoon soy sauce
  or tamari
- 2 teaspoon sesame oil

Instructions:

- Heat ½ tablespoon oil in a large skillet or wok over medium-high heat. Add the kale, salt and ¼ cup of water sautéing for 2-3 minutes until the kale starts to wilt. Simmer another 2-3 minutes to soften the kale. Transfer to a bowl.

- Add ½ tablespoon oil to the skillet or wok. When hot again, add the garlic, ginger and chopped green onion bulbs, stirring constantly to prevent burning the garlic. Sauté for 1-2 minutes. Add the red peppers and sauté another 2 minutes. Fold in the tuna pieces and stir-fry another 2 minutes until tuna is only slightly pink.

- Stir in the cooked greens, chopped scallion leaves, soy sauce and sesame oil. Serve as is or over a bed of rice or rice noodles.

CHICKEN STRAWBERRY SPINACH SALAD:

Ingredients:

- 2 ½ cups sliced strawberries, divided
- 1 shallot, peeled

- ¼ cup canola or grape seed oil
- ¼ teaspoon each sea salt and ground black pepper
- 2 ½ tablespoon apple cider vinegar
- 2 tablespoon honey
- 1 teaspoon poppy seeds
- 2 cups baby spinach
- 2 cups romaine lettuce, chopped
- 3 cups shredded rotisserie chicken
- ½ cup sliced almonds, toasted
- 1 small whole grain baguette, cut into slices
- 1 cup goat cheese

Directions:

- In a blender or food processor, blend ½ cup strawberries with the shallot. Transfer to a small bowl and whisk in ¼ cup canola or grape seed oil with ¼ teaspoon each salt and pepper and the next 3 ingredients (thought poppy seeds) in a small bowl. Set aside.

- Combine the remaining strawberries, spinach, and romaine in a large salad bowl. Add the chicken and vinaigrette; toss gently to coat. Sprinkle with sliced almonds. Serve immediately with whole

grain rolls and goat
cheese.

POACHED EGG IN AVOCADO:

Ingredients:

- 1 egg
- 1 avocado

Directions:

- Fill bowl with cold water and crack egg into water.

- Microwave on low for 2 minutes.

- Drain egg and set aside.

- Pit avocado and place egg in hole.

- Salt and pepper to taste.

FOIL-GRILLED APRICOT GLAZED SALMON:

Ingredients:

- 1 1/3 punds salmon fillets (wild salmon when available)
- ¼ teaspoon freshly ground black pepper
- 1 Tablespoon extra-virgin olive oil
- 1 clove garlic, minced
- 1/3 cup apricot fruit spread, 100 percent fruit

- 1 Tablespoon Dijon mustard
- ½ cup low-sodium vegetable broth

Directions:

- Preheat grill to medium heat.

- Pat salmon dry with a paper towel and cut into four equal servings. Season the skinless side of salmon

- Place each piece of salmon on a double layer of foil with skin side down. Fold the sides of the foil up so that the cooking liquid will not run out.

- In a small bowl, whisk together the rest of the ingredients. Pour the liquid over the four pieces of salmon so that the glaze is distributed equally.

- Seal each foil by folding as if you were wrapping a gift. Slide the foil packets onto the grill and close the lid.

- Cook until the salmon is cooked through, about 10 minutes. Let it rest for 2 minutes and then unwrap and serve salmon over a bed of This dish can be served

hot or at room
temperature.

STUFFED CHICKEN BREAST:

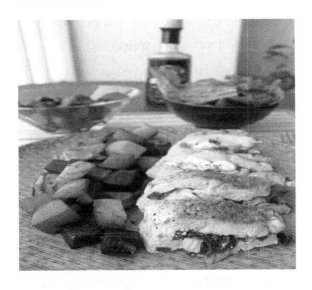

INGREDIENTS:

- 1 chicken breast
- 1 oz. low-fat mozzarella

- 1 artichoke heart (from a can)
- 1 tsp. sundried tomato, (chopped)
- 5 large basil leaves
- 1 clove garlic
- ¼ tsp. curry powder
- ¼ tsp. paprika
- Pinch of pepper

Directions:

- Preheat the oven to 365 F (185 C).

- About halfway up the chicken breast, cut a slit lengthwise to create a pocket for the filling.

- Chop up the mozzarella, artichoke, basil, tomato,

and garlic. Mix to combine.

- Stuff the mixture into the chicken breast where you created the pocket.

- Use a few toothpicks to close the chicken breast around the stuffing.

- Place the chicken breast on a baking sheet or aluminum foil and season it with pepper, curry powder, and paprika.

- Bake for around 20 minutes (depending on

the size of the chicken breast).

- Remove toothpicks and serve!

LOW CARB ZUCCHINI LASAGNA:

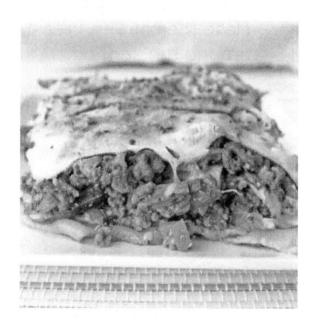

Ingredients:

- 16 oz. ground beef, (92% lean)
- 2 medium zucchini
- 4½ oz. onion
- 2 cloves garlic
- 1 serrano chili
- 3 tomatoes
- 5½ oz. mushrooms
- ½ cube Knorr chicken bouillon
- ½ cup shredded low-fat mozzarella
- 1 tsp. paprika
- 1 tsp. dried thyme
- 1 tsp. dried basil
- Salt & pepper
- Cooking spray

Directions:

- Use a julienne peeler to cut the zucchini into ½-

inch (1 cm) slices.
Sprinkle lightly with salt
and set aside for 10
minutes.

- Blot the zucchini slices
with a paper towel.
Either grill or broil them
in the oven for 3
minutes at high heat.

- After grilling or broiling,
place the zucchini on
paper towels (you want
to get as much of the
liquid out as possible).

- Cut off the ends of the
tomatoes and make an
X insertion on top. Place
in boiling water for a
few minutes, then pour
cold water over them

and peel off the skin. Alternatively, you could use canned tomatoes.

- Roughly chop onions, garlic, chili, peeled tomatoes, and mushrooms.

- Add a little cooking spray to a deep skillet and fry the garlic, onion, and chili for 1 min.

- Add the tomatoes and mushrooms to the skillet and sauté the vegetables for an additional 4 minutes. Then take them off the heat and set aside.

- Cook the beef with the paprika in the same skillet you used for the veggies until fully browned.

- Add the vegetables back into the skillet, then add the chicken bouillon and remaining spices. Allow the sauce to simmer for 25 minutes over low heat.

- Heat the oven to 375 degrees F (190 C).

- Line a small baking tray with parchment paper and use 1/3 of the zucchini to make a layer in the bottom. Put 1/3 of the meat sauce on top. Add another layer of zucchini and continue like this until you're out of sauce and zucchini.

- Spread shredded mozzarella on top and bake for 35 minutes.

- Take the lasagna out of the oven and allow to rest for 10 minutes before serving.

COCONUT CHICKEN SOUP:

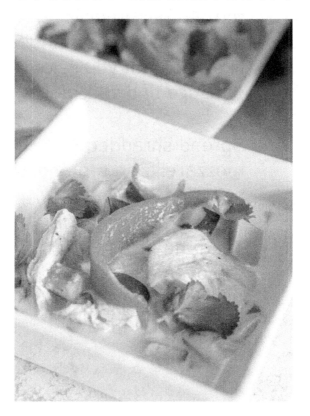

Ingredients:

- 1 lb. chicken breast, thinly sliced
- Salt & pepper, to taste

- 1 tbsp. coconut oil (or vegetable oil)
- 1 small onion, thinly sliced into half moons
- 2 garlic cloves, minced
- 1inch piece ginger, peeled and minced
- 1 medium zucchini, cut into quarters lengthwise and diced
- 0.75 lb. pumpkin, cubed into ½ inch pieces (1 cup)
- 1 red bell pepper, seeds removed and thinly sliced
- 1 small chili or jalapeño pepper, seeds removed and thinly sliced
- 14 oz. lite coconut milk (1 can)

- 2 cups chicken broth
- Juice of 1 lime
- Handful cilantro leaves

Directions:

- Season the sliced chicken breast generously with salt and pepper.

- In a large (5-6 quart) soup pot, heat the coconut oil over high heat and add the chicken breast. Stir-fry over high heat for 4-5 minutes, or until the chicken is no longer pink on the outside.

- Add the sliced onion, minced garlic, and

minced ginger. Continue to stir-fry for another 2-3 minutes.

- Add the diced zucchini and cubed pumpkin, then stir.

- Add the sliced bell pepper, sliced chili or jalapeño pepper, coconut milk, chicken broth, and lime juice. Give everything another good stir.

- Bring to a boil, then lower the heat, cover, and allow to simmer for about 20 minutes, or until the pumpkin is fully cooked.\Remove

from heat and season
with additional salt and
pepper, if desired.
Garnish with

BEEF FAJITAS:

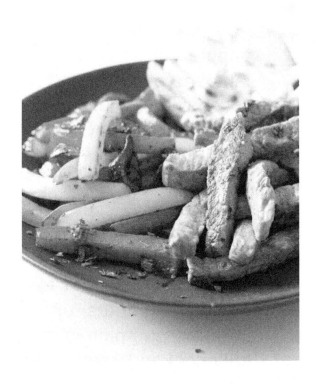

Ingredients:

- 1 lbs. beef stir-fry strips
- 1 medium red onion
- 1 red bell pepper
- 1 yellow bell pepper
- ½ tsp. cumin
- ½ tsp. chilli powder
- splash of oil
- Salt
- Pepper
- Juice of half a lime
- Freshly chopped cilantro (also called coriander)
- 1 avocado

Directions:

- Heat a cast-iron skillet over medium heat.

- Wash and deseed bell peppers, then slice

them into 1/4" (0.5 cm) thick long stripes. Set aside.

- Peel and slice red onion. Set aside.

- Once skillet is hot, add a splash of oil. When the oil is hot, add stir-fry strips in 2-3 batches. Make sure the strips don't touch each other.

- Salt and pepper each beef stir-fry batch generously in the pan. Cook for about 1 minute per side, then set aside on a plate and cover to keep warm.

- Once all the beef is cooked and set aside, add sliced onions and bell peppers to the remaining meat juice. Season with cumin and chili powder, then stir-fry until desired consistency.

- Transfer the veggies and beef stir-fry strips to a plate and serve with sliced avocado, a drizzle of lemon juice, and a sprinkle of fresh cilantro.

INSTANT POT CHICKEN CHILI:

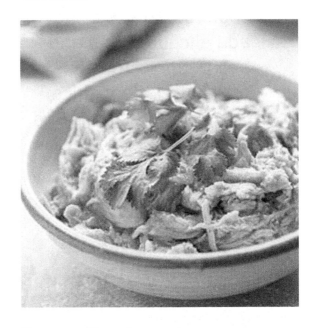

Ingredients:

- 1 tbsp. vegetable oil
- 1 yellow onion, diced
- 4 cloves garlic, minced
- 1 tsp. ground cumin
- 1 tsp. oregano

- 2 ½ lbs. chicken breasts, boneless & skinless
- 16 oz. salsa verde

Toppings

- 2 packages queso fresco (crumbled, or sour cream)
- 2 avocados, diced
- 8 radishes, chopped fine
- 8 springs cilantro (optional)

Directions:

- Set the Instant Pot to the sauté setting on medium.

- Add the vegetable oil.

- Add the onion and cook for 3 minutes, stirring frequently until the onion begins to soften.

- Add the garlic, and stir for another minute.

- Add the cumin and oregano and stir for another minute.

- Pour ½ of the salsa verde into the pot. Top with the chicken breasts and pour the remaining salsa verde over the chicken.

- Place the lid on the Instant Pot, turn the valve to "sealing," and select "manual". Set the timer for 10 minutes.

- Once the timer is up, let the pressure release naturally (will take 8-10 minutes).

- After the pressure has come down, open the lid, transfer the chicken to a medium bowl, and shred with a fork.

- Return the chicken to the pot and stir to combine with the rest of the ingredients.

SLOW COOKER SEAFOOD RAMEN:

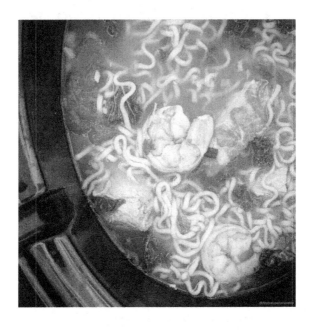

Ingredients:

* 64 oz broth (seafood, vegetable, or chicken

* 4–6 oz ramen

* 1 lb seafood

* 2 green onions, sliced

* 2 tbsp low-sodium soy sauce

* 2 tbsp rice vinegar

* 2 garlic cloves, minced

* 1/4 cup kale, chopped

* 1/2 lb tomatoes, sliced

* 1/4 tsp sesame oil

* 1 tsp salt

* 1/4 tsp pepper

* 1/8 tsp red pepper flakes

Directions:

- Add all ingredients except the seafood, kale

and ramen to the slow cooker. Stir to mix well.

- Cook on high for 2-3 hours, or low for 4-6 hours.

- Add seafood, kale & ramen and cook for an additional 15-30 minutes.

LOADED CAULIFLOWER:

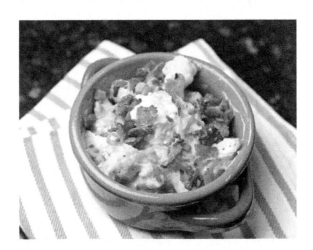

Ingredients:

- 1.25 lb cauliflower head, cut into florets
- 6 green onions, chopped into the green and white parts
- 2 tbsp butter
- 3 garlic cloves, minced
- 2 oz cream cheese
- 1/2 tsp sea salt
- 1/4 tsp black pepper
- 1.5 tsp ranch seasoning Mix, optional
- 3/4 c. organic heavy whipping cream
- 2 c. cheddar cheese, grated
- 4 slices sugar-free bacon, crumbled

- Olive oil for roasting the cauliflower
- Dollops of sour cream, optional

Directions:

- Preheat the oven to 425 degrees.

- Toss the cauliflower with ~2 Tbsp of olive oil then add it to a baking sheet. Roast the cauliflower on a baking sheet for 25 minutes. The cauliflower will get tender and some parts will brown up.

- While the cauliflower is roasting, make the cheese sauce: Add butter, the white parts of the green onions, and the garlic cloves to a skillet on medium heat. Sauté until the onions are translucent (~3 minutes).

- Add heavy cream, cream cheese, salt, ranch seasoning (if you're using it), and pepper to the skillet with the onions, garlic and butter. Turn the heat to medium low and continue to cook until the cream cheese is melted. Stir in 1.5 cups of the cheddar cheese to finish the cheese sauce.

- Mix the cheese sauce and the roasted cauliflower, then add it to a baking dish. Top it with the remaining cheddar cheese and roast for an additional 20 minutes, or until the cauliflower is tender.

- Top the baked cauliflower, with some dollops of sour cream, the green parts of the green onions, and the crumbled bacon.

QUICK AND EASY MONGOLIAN BEEF:

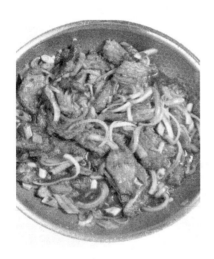

Ingredients:

- 1 lb flank steak thinly sliced against the grain
- 2 Tbsp cornstarch
- 2-4 Tbsp canola oil
- 1 yellow onion sliced

- 2 green onions chopped, green and white parts separated
- 4 garlic cloves chopped
- 1- inch ginger chopped
- ¼ c. low sodium soy sauce
- ¼ c. water
- 1 Tbsp hoisin sauce
- 3 Tbsp brown sugar
- Salt to taste

Directions:

- Cover the flank steak with cornstarch, making sure each piece is covered. Set aside.

- Heat the canola oil in a large skillet over medium-high heat.

Once the oil is hot, add
the flank steak to the
frying pan in a single
layer, making sure that
the pieces are not
touching. Cook for 1-2
minutes per side until
each side is browned.
Cook in batches until all
the flank steak is
cooked. Set aside.

- Add sliced yellow onion,
  whites of green onions,
  garlic, and ginger to the
  skillet and stir fry for
  about 3 minutes, until
  the onions are slightly
  softened but still have a
  little crunch. Add soy
  sauce, water, hoisin
  sauce, and brown sugar

and stir. Add steak back to the pan along with the green parts of the onions. Remove from heat and serve.

CARIBBEAN STEAMED FISH:

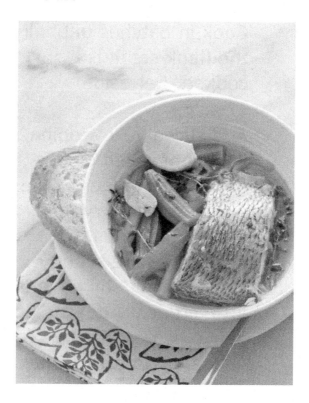

Ingredients:

- 2 lbs fish (porgy or snapper), cleaned and scaled
- Juice of 1 lime
- ½ tsp black pepper
- 1 tsp salt
- 3 cloves garlic – 2 sliced and 1 crushed
- About 15 sprigs thyme
- ½ Tbsp butter
- ½ Tbsp oil
- 2 carrots, thinly sliced
- 1 red pepper, thinly sliced
- 1 green pepper, thinly sliced
- 1 onion, thinly sliced
- 12 okra, ends cut off

- 1 hot pepper (scotch bonnet, habanero or wiri wiri), seeds removed
- 1 ½ cup water

DIRECTIONS:

- Season the fish with lime juice, crushed garlic, black pepper, salt and half of the thyme and set aside.

- In a large, wide heavy bottom pot over medium heat, add oil and butter. When butter has melted, sauté carrots, red and green pepper, and onion until it has softened, about 5 minutes.

- Add garlic slices and pepper and cook for just a minute or two. Add water and bring to a boil. Add fish to the pot. Spoon some of the vegetables on top of the fish. Add okra and the rest of the thyme.

- Cover the pot and lower the heat to simmer then cook for 15 minutes until the fish is done. Remove from heat and serve.

CRISPY POTATO TACOS:

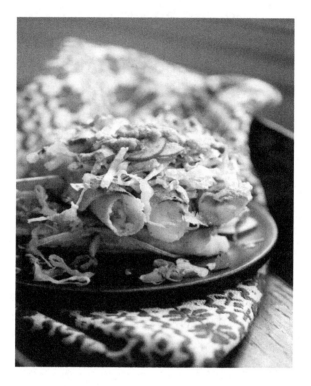

Ingredients:

- 12 corn tortillas
- 1 c. mashed potatoes
- 4 Tbsp of vegetable oil or avocado oil

- 4 long wooden skewers

To serve:

- Thinly sliced romaine lettuce or green cabbage
- Radishes thinly sliced
- Cilantro
- Guacamole
- Salsa verde.

Directions:

- Heat tortillas on a skillet for 10-15 seconds to make them pliable.

- Put a spoonful of mashed potatoes in the center of each tortilla and spread it along the tortilla. Roll the tortilla and put it on a long skewer. Repeat until you put three or four tacos on the skewer.

- Repeat with all the tortillas.

- In a frying pan over high heat put a tablespoon of oil and put three or four tacos, leave until golden brown, three to five minutes, turn and brown on the other side.

- Take out the tacos and put in a dish with a paper towel to absorb the excess oil.

- Repeat until all the tacos are done.

- To serve, put the crispy potato tacos on a plate and finish with the toppings. Enjoy immediately.

BLACK GARLIC, SESAME AND SHITAKE COD:

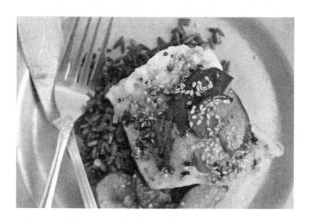

Ingredients:

- 2 Alaskan Cod filets, frozen
- 1 clove black garlic
- 2 Tbsp olive oil
- 1 tsp sesame seeds
- 1/2 c. dried shiitake, rehydrated

DIRECTIONS:

- Preheat your oven to 450F.

- Rinse frozen fish, pat dry with a paper towel, and place on a non-stick pan.

- In a small bowl, place black garlic and warm in

the microwave for 10 seconds.

- Mash the garlic clove and add olive oil and sesame seeds.

- Brush this mixture on frozen filets and sprinkle the mushrooms around the fish.

- Place in the oven for 12-15 minutes, depending on the thickness of the fish. If your filets are on the thick side, flip halfway through cooking.

- Serve alongside rice, your favorite salad, or whole grain.

SHRIMP LETTUCE WRAPS:

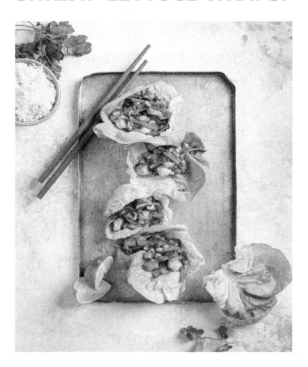

Ingredients:

- 1 head butter lettuce or romaine lettuce hearts
- ¼ c. low-sodium chicken broth
- 1 Tbsp hoisin sauce
- ½ Tbsp low-sodium soy sauce
- 1 tsp rice vinegar
- ¼ tsp Asian sesame oil
- 1 1/2 tsp chili garlic sauce
- ½ tsp cornstarch
- 1 Tbsp canola or avocado oil divided
- 30 grams' cashews little less than ¼ cup, coarsely chopped
- 6 oz shrimp deveined & cut into small cubes

- 1 large garlic clove minced
- 1/2 large red bell pepper seeded and diced
- 3 green onions the white and green parts, sliced
- ⅛ c. chopped cilantro
- 1 carrot shredded or cut into thin strips

Directions:

- Divide the lettuce into leaves and set aside.

- In a small bowl, whisk together the chicken broth, hoisin sauce, soy sauce, rice vinegar, sesame oil, chili garlic

sauce, and cornstarch.
Set aside.

- In a medium skillet,
  heat ½ Tbsp canola or
  avocado oil over
  medium-high heat until
  almost smoking.

- Add the shrimp and stir-
  fry until browned. About
  2 minutes. Transfer the
  shrimp to a plate and
  discard any juices from
  the pan.

- In the same skillet, heat
  the other ½ tablespoon
  of oil over medium-high
  heat.

- Add the garlic, bell pepper, green onions, and carrots.

- Stir fry until tender-crisp, about 2 minutes.

- Return the shrimp to the pan and add the cashews and cilantro. Add the soy-sauce mixture and stir-fry until the shrimp is thoroughly cooked. About 3 minutes.

- Spoon the shrimp mixture evenly onto lettuce leaves.

GRILLED CHICKEN AND VEGETABLE SHISH KEBABS:

Ingredients:

- 2 Tbsp Better Than Bouillon roasted chicken base
- 2 lb boneless chicken breasts
- 8 oz cubed pineapples
- 1 red bell pepper
- 1 green bell pepper
- 1 orange bell pepper
- 1 whole zucchini
- 2 tsp oregano
- 2 tsp black pepper
- 2 tsp paprika.

For the teriyaki pineapple sauce

- 1/2 c. low-sodium soy sauce
- 2 tsp minced garlic
- 2 tsp Sesame Oil
- 2 Tbsp fresh pineapple juice
- 2 tsp cornstarch
- 1 tsp black pepper
- 1/4 tsp Himalayan salt
- 1/4 tsp garlic powder
- 2 Tbsp brown sugar

Directions:

- Begin by starting your fire on the grill and allow the temperature to reach 350 degrees.

- Cut your chicken breast into cubes and place into a large bowl.

Season chicken with oregano, black pepper and paprika then rub ingredients into the chicken.

- Add Better Than Bouillon roasted chicken base to the chicken. Mix together well then set to the side.

- Remove the stem and seeds from each of the bell peppers and cut into large pieces. Chop the zucchini into slices.

- Place each ingredient individually onto the skewers in desired order.

- Place each chicken and veggie skewer onto the grill. Grill for 4 minutes each side. Remove from heat.

- For the sauce, add all ingredients into a small cooking pan on medium/high heat until it begins to bubble then lower heat to simmer and cook for 8 minutes and remove from heat and allow to cool.

- Serve immediately.

ZUCCHINI PIZZA BOATS:

Ingredients:

- 4 medium zucchini

- ¼ tsp kosher salt
- 1 c. pizza sauce — or similar prepared marinara sauce
- 1 ¼ c. shredded mozzarella cheese — or a blend of shredded mozzarella and provolone
- 1 tsp Italian seasoning
- ¼ - ½ tsp crushed red pepper flakes — optional
- ¼ c. mini pepperoni — or mini turkey pepperoni or regular-size pepperoni, sliced into quarters
- 2 tsp freshly ground Parmesan

- 2 tsp chopped fresh basil, thyme, or other fresh herbs

Directions:

- Place a rack in the center of your oven. Preheat the oven to 375 degrees F. Lightly coat a rimmed baking sheet or 9x13-inch baking dish with nonstick spray.

- Halve each zucchini lengthwise. With a small spoon or melon baller, gently scrape out the center zucchini flesh and pulp, leaving a border of about 1/3 inch on all sides. Arrange the zucchini shells on the

baking sheet. Sprinkle
the insides of the
zucchini with salt.

- Spoon the pizza sauce
  into each shell, dividing
  it evenly. You may need
  a little more or less,
  depending upon the size
  of your zucchini. Put a
  generous amount, but
  don't feel like you need
  to fill it all the way to
  the very top.

- Sprinkle the mozzarella
  over the top, then
  evenly sprinkle with
  Italian seasoning and
  red pepper flakes (if
  using). Scatter on the
  pepperoni and any other

desired toppings. Last, sprinkle with Parmesan.

- Bake for 15 to 20 minutes, until the cheese is hot and bubbly and the zucchini is tender. If desired, switch the oven to broil and cook the zucchini for 2 to 3 additional minutes, until the cheese is lightly browned. Remove from the oven and sprinkle with chopped fresh basil. Serve immediately.

CREAMY GLUTEN-FREE TOMATO PASTA:

Ingredients:

- 3 Tbsp olive oil (divided)
- ½ c. diced white onion
- 1 tsp minced garlic
- 10 oz gluten free pasta
- 8 oz canned Italian stewed tomatoes (drained)
- ¼ c. paleo mayo
- 1 egg yolk
- ¼ tsp each kosher salt and black pepper
- Optional ½ tsp crushed red pepper flakes
- Fresh basil and cracked pepper

Directions:

- In a small pan, sauté onions and garlic in 1 tbsp olive until fragrant, about 2 minutes. Once they are almost cooked, set aside.

- In a large pot, cook your gluten free pasta according to directions.

- Drain, rinse the pasta, and place pasta back into pot. Keep on low heat.

- Mix in the remaining 2 tbsp olive oil and mix well. Mix gently.

- In a separate bowl, whisk together the mayo and egg yolk. Add this mix to your pot with the pasta, coating

until creamy. Gently
mix in the sauteed
onion/garlic.

- Toss the pasta with the
tomatoes, kosher salt
and pepper.

- Stir gently over low to
medium low heat until
creamy and combined.

- If using a cooked
protein, add it in here.

- Plate pasta into bowls.
Garnish with fresh basil
and cracked pepper.

MEXICAN SALAD WITH CHIPOTLE SHRIMP:

Ingredients:

- 2 lb raw jumbo shrimp, peeled and cleaned (tail on or off)
- 8 c. chopped kale
- 4 ears corn on the cob, shucked
- 15 oz can black beans, drained
- 1-pint grape or cherry tomatoes, halved
- 1 whole ripe avocado, peeled and chopped
- 2-3 whole chipotle peppers in adobo sauce
- 7 Tbsp fresh lime juice, divided
- ¼ c. olive oil
- ¼ c. mayonnaise
- 2 Tbsp honey
- 3 cloves garlic
- ½ tsp salt

Directions:

- Preheat the grill to medium heat. To a blender jar, add the chipotle peppers, 4 tablespoons of lime juice, olive oil, garlic, and salt. Cover and puree until smooth.

- Measure out 3 tablespoons of the chipotle puree and save it for the dressing. In a medium bowl, mix the shrimp and the remaining marinade, until well coated.

- In a separate small bowl, mix the 3 tablespoons of chipotle puree, 3 tablespoons lime juice, mayonnaise, and honey. Whisk until smooth. Then taste, and salt and pepper as needed.

- Prep all the veggies. Set out a large salad bowl. Add the kale. Then toss it with the dressing until well coated. (I like to massage the dressing into the kale by hand.) Then add in the black beans, tomatoes, and avocado.

- Place the shrimp and corn cobs on the grills. *If your shrimp are small they will fall

through the grates.
Either use a grill basket,
or place them on a
piece of foil. Grill the
shrimp for 3-5 minutes
until pink. Grill the corn
for 8-10 minutes
rotating every 2
minutes.

- Once the corn is cool
enough to handle, cut it
off the cobs and add it
to the salad. Then toss
in the shrimp and serve.

ALKALINE WARRIOR CHIA:

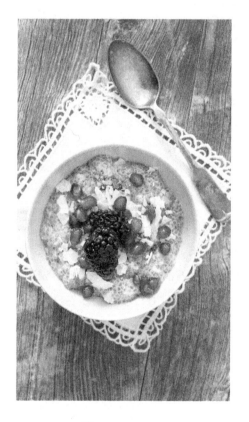

Ingredients:

- 1 cup unsweetened almond or coconut milk
- 4 tbsp. of chia seeds
- ½ tsp. vanilla
- ½ tsp. cinnamon
- 1 tbsp. unsweetened shredded coconut flakes
- ¼ cup chopped nuts (almonds, cashews or hemp seeds).

Directions:

- The night before, combine milk and chia seeds in a mason jar. Add vanilla, cinnamon and chopped nuts. Cover with lid and shake the mixture until it's combined. Refrigerate overnight. The next morning, shake or stir the

mixture and divide into
2-3 bowls. Top with
optional fresh fruit,
coconut shreds or more
chopped nuts.

ALMOND BUTTER CRUNCH BERRY SMOOTHIE:

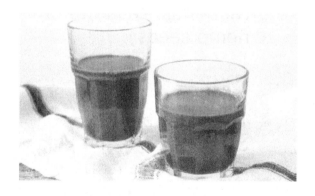

Ingredients:

- 2 cups fresh spinach
- 2 cups almond milk, unsweetened
- 1 cup of any of the following (frozen mixed

berries, strawberries or
grapes)
- 1 banana (peeled and
frozen)
- 4 tbsp. raw almond
butter
- 1 tbsp. chia.

Directions:

Blend spinach and almond
milk first. Then add
remaining ingredients except
chia, and blend. Add chia
once all is smooth – then
blend on a very low speed to
mix. If you don't have a
variable speed blender, mix
chia in with the rest of the
ingredients by hand. Let sit
for a few minutes for the
chia seeds to expand, then
enjoy.

KALE PESTO PASTA:

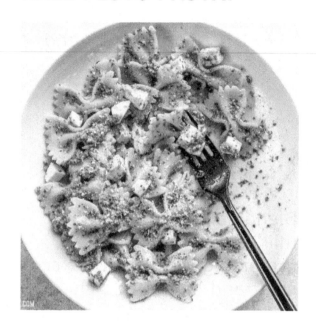

Ingredients:

- 1 bunch kale
- 2 cups fresh basil
- 1/4 cup extra virgin olive oil
- 1/2 cup walnuts
- 2 limes, fresh squeezed

Sea salt and pepper.

- 1 zucchini, noodled (spiralizer)
- Optional: garnish with sliced asparagus, spinach leaves, and tomato.

Directions:

The night before, soak walnuts to improve absorption. Put all ingredients in a blender or food processor, and blend until you get a cream consistency. Add to zucchini noodles and enjoy!

MANGO COCONUT GRANOLA:

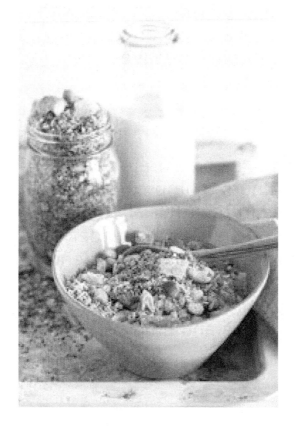

Packaged granola is normally loaded together with sugar, preservatives, in addition to other unsavory what won't accurately enable you to recharge. The remedy? Choose your own.

This specific easy recipe includes *fiber rich foods, nuts, dried up fruit, somewhat regarding oil, and a new touch of walnut syrup.*

Anybody else swallowing antibiotics or pain reducers? Figured. I'm inside a snowy metropolis; the sky is usually colorless. I'm dry-coughing my way to be able to the ending associated with an infection, rasping like an inveterate cigar smoker (or the spawn associated with Tom Waits). I would really like to be capable to complain for winter but I possess no real trigger. This is a more truthful picture: noon exceeded by me nevertheless lounging in mattress, with coffee with fresh fruit, and booking my springtime vacation. After this particular? I don't understand. I could spend the day watching films and reading poems about snow. Yes, life is raw. I really like wallowing.

This particular has been another winter for me personally, psychologically at minimum. I think I have made some type of tentative serenity with cold temperature. I even look for chilly walks round the town. I fell into a subtle rhythm of yoga, art, writing--rinse, again. The cold is present, but it feels irrelevant. All this time spent indoors writing, reading, and working quietly on projects has shifted my perspective on food preparation, too. I'm working on creating leaner and easier healthy recipes. Simpler meals. Less overwrought complexity and multi-step endeavors. (Which isn't to say that I am now about preparing something like Ottolenghi's 5-hours simmered chickpeas--

delicious and entirely worth every minute). Basically, I feel more balanced and relaxed on the whole this winter.

In the spirit of promoting optimal balance, if you've made some sort of vague resolution to clean up your game in this book, here is the cheerful and thoroughly clean breakfast idea: ***manga coconut cluster granola with coconut yogurt and fresh mangoes***. Mangoes are one of my absolute favorite fruits and the combination of dried and fresh mangoes is bright and sweet, playing off slightly different taste notes.

Pro tip:

Prepare huge batches of granola and then stockpile it in the freezer forever. No need to defrost--the fruit will harden somewhat but will obtain room temperature within minutes. As always, feel free to substitute other types of fruit or dairy yogurt for the coconut version.

Ingredients:

*2 cups woefully outdated rolled oats;

*5 cup raw cashews, chopped;

*1/2 glass unsweetened shredded or flaked coconut;

*1/4 cup sliced walnuts;

*1/2 tbsp. flax seeds (optional);

*3 tbsp. maple viscous syrup;

*2 tbsp. organic and natural virgin unrefined coconut oil;

*1/2 teaspoon ground ginger;

*25 tsp ground cinnamon;

*1/4 tsp the sea salt;

*1 egg white;

*2 cups sliced dried fruit: organic and natural apricots, dried mangoes;

To serve: fresh sliced mango, fat free yogurt.

Directions:

*Preheat the cooker to 325 Fahrenheit;

*Combine the first five ingredients in a huge bowl. Heat the coconut oil and maple syrup in a microwave or on the stovetop until the oil has just melted. Whisk in the spices and sea salt. Toss with the oats and nuts until the mixture is evenly coated;

*Whisk an egg white in a small bowl until frothy. Stir into the granola mixture. Spread the granola on a big baking sheet in an even layer;

*Bake for about 20 to 25 minutes. Halfway through the baking time, carefully turn sections of the granola over with a spatula, but do not break it up too much. When the granola is golden brown, remove from the oven and carefully stir in the sliced dried fruit. Allow the granola to cool completely. It will harden as it cools;

*Serve with yogurt and fresh fruit. Store in the cupboard in an airtight container or in the freezer in an airtight freezer bag.

Note: I bake the granola at a low temperature of about 300/325 F, because my oven chars everything. With a weaker oven, you may boost the temperature to 350 F. For larger clumps, do not stir the granola mix too much after adding the egg white and during/after baking. Conversely, for a flakier granola, stir well to break up the clusters.

BERRIES

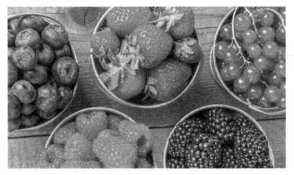

Grab fruits for an effective dose of illness fighting antioxidants. The color associated with berries comes through the pigment anthocyanin, an antioxidant that will helps neutralize "free radicals" (cell-damaging molecules) that can assist result in chronic illnesses, including cancer plus heart problems. Berries, especially cranberries, may furthermore help ward away urinary tract bacterial infections.

Have a cup of berries each day, as a snack; atop your cereal or yogurt; in muffins, salads, or smoothies; or as frozen treats.

These bite-sized fruit favorites are check filled with antioxidants, recognized to boost immunity and stave away life-threatening disease. They will help you age gracefully as nicely. A 2012 study from Harvard College found that in least one helping of blueberries or two servings of strawberries each week may reduce the risk of cognitive decline in old adults.

RAISINS:

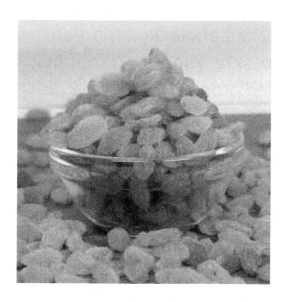

Raisins are a tasty natural snack that can be eaten on their own or added to a variety of recipes, such as oatmeal raisin cookies. In addition to being so versatile, they're also simple to make.

Serving Suggestion: Suggested storage containers for air-dried raisins include Mylar bags, Tupperware, and glass canning jars with an oxygen absorber. Homemade Raisins made this way and saved in an airtight container can be saved in a cool, dry place for several months.

Ingredients:

- 500 gams green grapes
- 3-4 water for boiling.

Directions:

- Collect all the required ingredients.
- Take green grapes and remove the larger stems from your grapes.
- Rinse the grapes under running water to wash them.
- Wash thoroughly for 3-4 times.
- Take enough water in a deep pan for blanching.
- Before drying your grapes, you'll want to blanch them. You can skip this step if you want, but blanching your grapes first softens the skins and helps them dry evenly. And it

only takes a minute. Do not boil the water is just heat it.
- When the water starts heating, drop the grapes.
- After 2-3 minutes, the grapes will starts floating above the water.
- When the grapes will boil over and the crack has come in them too. Switch off the flame.
- Do not over boil the grapes.
- As soon as the grapefruit starts floating and all our grape exploded from the

center, take them out
from the water.

- Take out the grapes
from water using sieve
or spoon.
- Let them cool for 5-7
minutes.
- Take a plate/tray or
basket and spread
cheesecloth/kitchen
towel/cotton cloth.
- Spread the grapes over
the cloth.
- Place the tray outside in
a dry sunny place. Take
the tray inside in the
night if it is foggy. Every
day keep it out in the
morning and take it
inside in the night. Keep
rotating the fruit for

even exposure to the sun. It takes around 1 to 2 days depending on the strength of the sun rays.

- Once the grapes have dried to the point of becoming raisins, take the tray inside and place the raisins in an airtight container. Store the container in a cool place or refrigerate.

Notes:

- Over-ripe grapes will take longer to dry and may rot before drying. It's preferable to have slightly under-ripe, yet sweet, grapes.

- Watch for dampness or rot. If a few grapes go bad, remove them immediately from the tray and spread close by fruit out to dry. Remember that drying grapes will shrivel up and get small, not turn to mush and rot.
- Professionals often create raisins by dangling bunches of fruit from the string or even wire and enabling them to dried out. This is tougher than employing a toned tray but functions better because the fresh fruit

has maximum
atmosphere exposure.

FATTY FISH:

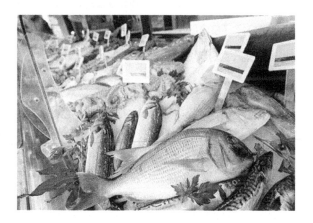

Omega-3 fatty acids are
usually abundant in seafood
like salmon plus tuna,
disease battling foods that
may help lower fats of blood
and prevent bloodstream
clots associated along with
heart disease.

Consuming a diet wealthy in fatty seafood can help slow up the risk of heart problems.

There's another advantage to eating foods containing salmon or even tuna: you'll decrease your potential consumption of saturated body fat from higher-fat entrees.

Fire up the particular grill or place your fish underneath the broiler for the quick, tasty, plus heart-healthy meal.

GREEN JUICE:

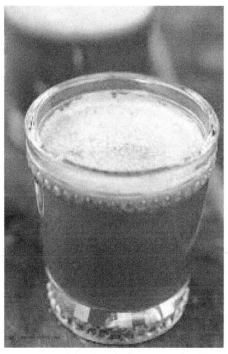

Juice one-inch each fresh

turmeric and ginger, one

handful each spinach and

kale, one cucumber, one cup

214

filtered water. Drink half,
and save the other half.

MEDITERRANEAN SEA
BREAKFAST TOSTADAS:

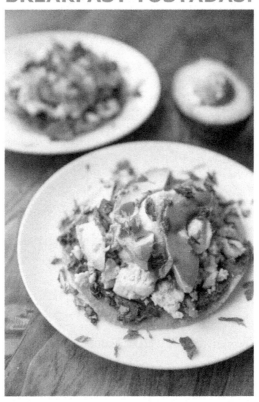

This might sound strange, but top a crisp tortilla with red pepper hummus, scrambled eggs, fresh tomatoes, cokes, and feta cheese and you've got one of the better unlikely breakfasts on the web.

Rich and creamy, fresh, and saline flavors blend to make this protein-rich breakfast stick with you.

Mediterranean **BREAKFAST** time Tostadas are a quick and healthy breakfast recipe that will fill you up and gas you during the day. Crispy tostadas are split with creamy red pepper hummus, screwed up eggs, veggies and feta for a well-rounded breakfast stuffed with bold Greek tastes!

So, I am completely obsessed with tostadas and this breakfast one just made it to the top of record. I actually do this for breakfast time ever single day until I went out of tostadas. If it was not breakfast time, we would just miss the eggs and make this as a satisfying treat. It is that good people! At first I wasn't all that sure how eggs and hummus would pair, but let me inform you, if you have not tried it yet, you are really missing out. This protein loaded breakfast is where it is at!

Evidently this is the time where people learn to loose grip using their New Year's resolutions. Is that you? Well, if you are sensation your strength sliding on your promise to eat better, this healthy breakfast time tostada is the perfect thing to truly get you back on monitor. Everybody knows the significance of eating breakfast, and if you choose it this delicious, you won't seem like you are sacrificing something!

Ingredients:

* 4 tostadas;

* 1/2 chemical. Roasted chili peppers hummus;

* 1/2 c. red pepper, diced;

* 0.5 c. green onions, chopped;

* 8 ovum beaten;

* 1/2 chemical. skim milk.

Steps:

* In a huge non-stick skillet over medium heat, add the red peppers and cook for 2 - 3 minutes until melted.

* Add the ovum, milk, garlic natural powder, oregano and eco-friendly onions to the

skillet, constantly mixing until egg white wines are no lengthier translucent (about 2 minutes).

* Top each tostada with hummus, eggs mixture, cucumber, tomatoes& feta. Serve immediately.

* 0.5 tsp. garlic natural powder;

* 1/2 tsp. oregano;

* 1/2 c. cucumber, seeded and cut;

* 1/2 c. tomato vegetables, diced;

* 1/4 chemical. feta crumbled;

* A few Avocado toasts together with charred tomatoes, garlic herb shrimp, and toast eggs.

This ramped-up take on ova and toast is usually a guest-worthy collation dish. Slather pieces of whole grain bread toasted with avocado and to the top 'elm with charred tomato plants, garlic shrimp, in addition to fried (or poached) eggs.

Who will not be thrilled to get served that from Sunday brunch?

I want to speak about camping in addition to

avocado toast. For the reason that order.

This avocado toast may be the jugs, and it must be shared immediately. Which, friends, is the reason why you are considering Avocado Toasts with Charred Tomato vegetables, Garlic Shrimp and to Fried Eggs as opposed to some type of gourmet warm dog situation.

This may end up being one of the most epic variation of avocado bread toasted ever. (And I actually say that together with authority because we eat some edition of avocado toasted bread at least 4 times in 7 days.) A great piece of grilled bread topped along with creamy avocado will be heavenly, but include charred tomatoes, rapidly sautéed garlicky shrimp with lemon and herbs, a completely cooked fried egg cell, and a nice sprinkling of Parmesan? FLAVOR BOMB. I mean, this is the avocado toast of your wildest dreams, people.

I know you're going to think this is a lot of effort for avocado toast, but bear with me. With a little organization, you can pull this thing off in about 20 minutes, and it is worth every single second. And, these toasts can be eaten *ANY TIME OF THE DAY,* and they're definitely impressive enough to serve to guests. I'm imagining them at an outdoor summer brunch with a bottle of light rosé. Yes? **Yes!**

Now that I think about it, I could totally make this avocado toast while camping, and I just might. Sure, it will take me a couple of extra minutes with only one pan and a camp stove, but let's be real, I've got nothing but time out in the particular "wild."

GARLIC:

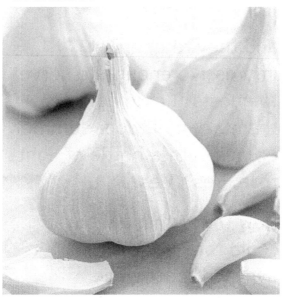

From a Pennsylvania banquet celebrating centenarians final spring, Nancy Fisher, 107, attributed the girl long life in order to her faith... plus her passion regarding garlic.

Fisher might be on in order to something, however:

Research have found that will phytochemicals in garlic clove can halt the particular formation of dangerous chemicals in your body, plus that women that consume more garlic have got lower risk associated with certain colon malignancies.

SPINACH-STUFFED SWEET POTATO:

For any hearty, healthy *LUNCH* time that comes with each other inside a jiffy, appear no further. Roast a sweet potato (if you're brief on time, take it in the particular microwave for seven to 10 minutes) after which fill this with sautéed spinach, kale, and new avocado, drizzled along with zesty tahini, turmeric, and lemon dressing up. Yum!

When a person starts referring in order to your fridge because "the cheese refrigerator," it will be both an indicator that will you're living your own best life, which your diet can perhaps make use of a minor tune up. These types of past two several weeks, I and my friends have been consuming our way via Paris, and because the previous statement indicates, it is often a deliciously hedonistic time therefore far. Following a flutter of baguettes, Contigu butter, squab (or pigeon, as it may be called here), wine beverages, chocolates, pâté, macarons, steak tartare, in addition to the aforementioned mozzarella cheese, my body is usually practically shouting for a leafy-greens-heavy dinner (or two).

At present, I can't obtain this spinach-, kale-, and avocado- capped baked sweet potato out of the head. Overlooking these types of pictures when I create, my mouth will be watering in the manner that will it normally might while gazing in a slice of cherry pie, a bloody steak, or the cheesy gratin. For valid reason: our own bodies are very good at informing us what these people need; moreover, this particular recipe provides within a major way.

Ingredients:

- For the sweet potato:

- 1 medium sweet potato

- 1/2 tablespoon coconut oil

- 1/2 teaspoon kosher salt

- Pinch of cayenne

- 1 cup baby spinach

- 1 cup torn (dribbled) kale leaves

- 1/4 avocado, diced

- Thinly-sliced scallions, for garnish

- Chopped cilantro, for garnish

For the turmeric dressing:

- 1 and 1/2 teaspoons tahini

- 1/4 teaspoon turmeric

- Juice of 1 lemon

- 1 teaspoon coconut oil, melted

- 1/2 garlic clove, minced

- Kosher salt, to taste

Directions:

1. Preheat the oven to 350°F.

2. Wash any dirt off of the sweet potato, then prick all over with a fork. Wrap in tinfoil then roast on a quarter-sheet pan for 45 minutes-1 hour, or until tender.

3. Meanwhile, make the dressing: whisk together all dressing ingredients until emulsified. Season to taste with salt.

4. Once the particular sweet potato will be tender, remove it associated with the

oven. Reduce the sweet spud in half

5. Heat the coconut oil in a huge skillet over medium-high heat. Add the particular spinach, kale, sodium, and cayenne, putting to coat within the melted essential oil. Cook, stirring regularly, until the vegetables are wilted, but nonetheless bright in colour.

6. Top every half of the particular sweet potato along with half of the particular cooked greens, diced avocado, scallions, and cilantro. Drizzle along with dressing and consume immediately.

OLIVE OIL

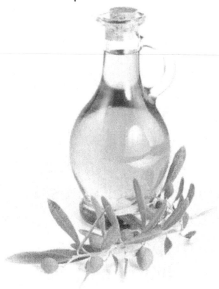

Since delightful as this is healthy, this particular monounsaturated "good fat" is well identified for its heart-health and longevity advantages. Studies also display that olive essential oil can also be linked in order to brain into the malignancy prevention. Strive for 2 tablespoons per day.

QUINOA BURRITO BOWL:

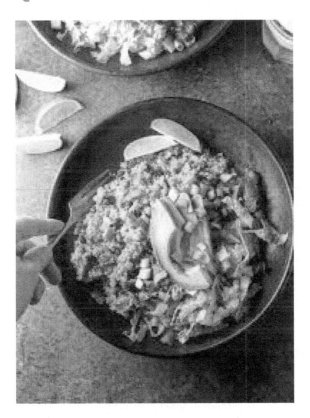

Ingredients:

- 1 cup quinoa (or brown rice)
- 2 15-oz cans of black or adzuki beans
- 4 green onions (scallions), sliced
- 2 limes, fresh juiced
- 4 garlic cloves, minced
- 1 heaping tsp. cumin
- 2 avocados, sliced
- small handful of cilantro, chopped.

Directions:

- Cook quinoa or rice. While cooking, warm beans over low heat. Stir in onions, lime juice, garlic and cumin and let flavors combine for 10-15 minutes. When quinoa is done

cooking, divide into
individual serving
bowls. Top with beans,
avocado and cilantro.

Studies indicates that
cruciferous veggies like this
a single contain nutrients,
this kind of as fiber,
supplement C, and folate,
that can assist you cheat loss
of life. And that's most likely
the case whether or not
you've already got a close
contact: A study through
Vanderbilt University
discovered that breast
malignancy survivors in
Shanghai in china who ate a
lot more cruciferae—
specifically of the particular
turnip, cabbage, plus bok

choy range popular in China—had lower risks associated with death or malignancy recurrence throughout the research period.

POP SUGAR|

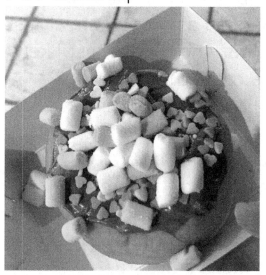

The Natural Food Globe

Buzzle

Eat healthy, remain healthy!

Ingredients:

* 4 tablespoon Chia Seed products

* 1. 25 mugs Milk Sugar (optional)

* Garnish (feel liberated to use seasonal fruits and nuts of your own choice)

* Apple Slices;

* Banana slices;

* Blueberries;

* Peach Slices;

* Sliced up Almonds;

* Raisins;

* Mint simply leaves;

Directions:

* Within a little bowl, include the chia seed products and pour the particular milk;

* Mix nicely having a fork. Location it within the fridge for at the very least 15-20 minutes. I actually mix the chia seeds with whole milk through the night and employ the soaked seed in the morning hours;

* After the chia seed are soaked, put sugar and added milk in accordance with your current taste;

* Transfer typically the contents to 2 providing bowls, add chopped up (seasonal) along with almonds.

That is super an easy task to make this vegetarian: substitute the whole milk with almond whole milk or soy whole milk.

You can even Vanilla fact, rose essence or perhaps cardamom to flavor the chia pudding.

DAIRY:

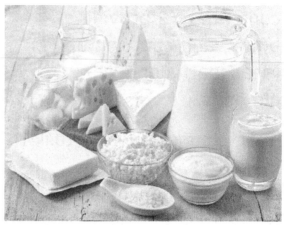

Dairy foods are not only the best food source of dietary calcium, but also have plenty of protein, vitamins (including vitamin D), and minerals -- key to fighting the disease osteoporosis. Having three daily servings of low-fat dairy products, as well as doing weight-bearing exercise, to help keep bones strong. (If you can't tolerate dairy, other calcium-containing foods include legumes; dark green leafy vegetables such as kale, broccoli, and collards; and calcium-fortified soy products, juices, and grains.)

Beyond strong bones, dairy may also help you lose weight. Research is ongoing, but a few studies have shown that three daily servings of dairy -- as part of a calorie-controlled diet -- may help decrease belly fat and enhance weight loss.

Low-fat dairy foods make excellent snacks because

they contain both carbohydrates and protein.

Dairy foods are perfect snacks for diabetics and everybody else because [they help] maintain blood sugars levels.

Whip upward a smoothie along with low-fat milk or even yogurt, a dash of orange fruit juice, along with a handful associated with berries to have a zestful meal substitute or even anytime snack.

AVOCADO:

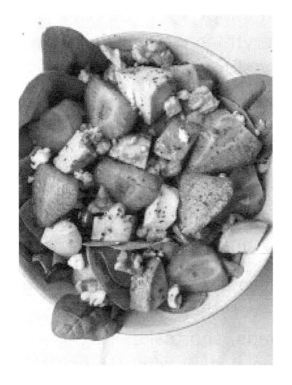

This salad will be the
associated with new. With
baby kale, strawberries,
avocado, red-colored onion,
cheese (because always
cheese), and sliced almonds

tossed in a homemade honey and poppy seed dressing. it's everything we could want in a healthy salad.

And you'd better believe that sweet advertising has worked on me...every time. Love me some good strawberries when they're in season!

In the past, I've tossed them in everything from salsas to salads, shortcakes to cheesecakes, smoothies to sangrias, and everything in between. But every year, my inaugural formula for strawberry time of year is always the particular same — this particular classic

Strawberry Avocado Spinach Salad along with Poppy Seed Dressing. This was one associated with the initial green salads that I discovered to like (and make) way back again in my picky-eating days, but still proceeds to be one of my personal favorite fairly sweet and simple fashion back recipes to create each spring.

In order to start, commence simply by hulling and halving a pint associated with ripe, red bananas. (I know it is almost impossible not really to just take these babies correct in your mouth area.

But keep in mind that, they will be worthwhile within the salad.)

Then, blend them with the rest of your ingredients. The list of specifics here is actually pretty flexible — you can go with lots of fresh baby spinach (or whatever greens you'd like), crumbled blue cheese (or any soft cheese), toasted almonds (or any nuts), and thinly-sliced red onion. But the non-negotiable is a huge, ripe, creamy avocado. Got to have typically the avocado.

Then within just minutes, this vivid and beautiful early spring salad will end up being yours to reveal and enjoy! It may be sweet, it's rich and creamy, it's crunchy, it may be tangy — it may be basically everything an individual can ask for in a good salad, if you ask me. ;)

Feel free to add in some grilled chicken or another protein if you'd like. Or if you'd like to make it a little heartier, I also love tossing in some chilled cooked faro or quinoa too. However, you make it, I hope you enjoy it!

Ingredients:

- 6 cups fresh child spinach

- 1 pint strawberries, hulled plus sliced

- 1 avocado, peeled, pitted plus diced (or you are able to double this in order to 2 avocados!)

- 4 ounces crumbled blue cheese (or goat cheese or even feta)

- 1/4 mug sliced almonds, done

- Half a little red-colored onion, thinly sliced up.

Poppy seed Dressing Components:

- 1/3 cup avocado oil (or olive oil)

- 3 Tablespoons apple cider white vinegar

- 2 tablespoons darling

- 1 tablespoon poppy seeds

- pinch associated with ground dry mustard (optional)

- fine ocean salt and freshly-cracked black pepper.

Directions:

Throw all ingredients with each other with your preferred amount of dressing up until combined. Function immediately.

To Create the Poppy Seed Dressing up:

Whisk almost all ingredients together till combined. Add the pinch of sodium and pepper, or even more to flavor.

Just how to prevent center disease, the most significant killer in the USA, in line with the latest report through the National Middle of Health Stats? Eat more meals that help maintain your heart healthful, like avocados plus others already upon this list, plus improve your chances of an extended lifestyle. Avocados can reduce your LDL "bad" cholesterol while increasing your HDL "good" levels, and they will help

your body absorb heart-
healthy vitamins like beta-
carotene and lycopene.

TOMATOES:

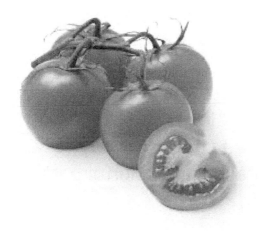

These red-hot fruits of
summer are bursting with
flavor and lycopene -- an
antioxidant that may help
protect against some

cancers. Additionally, they deliver a large quantity of vitamins The and C, potassium, and phytochemicals.

Take pleasure in tomatoes raw, prepared, sliced, chopped, or even diced included in any kind of meal or treat. Stuff a tomato half with kale and add roughly grated cheese for any fantastic and colorful part dish.

Lycopene is also an essential nutrient in the fight against cancer—the second leading cause of death in the United States. And there's no better source than rosy red tomatoes. Eating them cooked, in pasta sauce, tomato soup, or chutney, actually increases the amount of carcinogen-fighting carotenoids your body is able to absorb.

VEGETABLE QUINOA BITES:

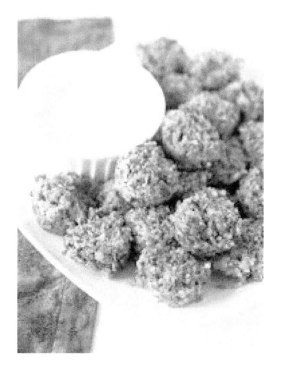

This snack is perfect for the 3 p. m. *(LUNCH)* workday munchies. These little protein-filled nuggets are made of quinoa, spinach, and shredded carrots, baked with eggs and cheddar cheese. That'll keep you full until mealtime.

If you are familiar with the food, then you have had to have seen these little bites making their way around the blogosphere. Genius, I have to say. A genius appetizer for the health-conscious. Super Bowl, anyone? Anyways, the first time I saw these was on Pinterest, then the food photography websites, and I knew I would be adding them to my ever-growing listing of "must-dos".

I've already talked about the health advantages of quinoa, but if you've got a box or bag of quinoa on hand, some leftover veggies to get rid of, and maybe a little bit of cheese on hand, then you've got an easy, savory, and bite-sized appetizer ready in less than 20 minutes.

I had ironically made quinoa for a little veggie dish the night before and was wondering what to do with the leftovers. I had cooked a lot of associated with the stuff to be able to remove the package create room within my pantry, therefore I had specifically 2 cups associated with cooked quinoa prepared to go. I had formed a few arbitrary carrots, some new spinach, and a few shallots available, as well. The beauty associated with this recipe will be its versatility within what you can include in to it. Peas? Probably. Corn? Probably. Him? Hopefully. I simply tossed the vegetables within my food processor chip and was great to go. And, as far because cheese goes, I added in certain razor-sharp cheddar in due to the fact I was from Parmesan. As lengthy as you may bind it almost all along with those ovum, my answer is adding because many veggies within as possible.

With regard to serving, I dropped them in Farm dressing. Probably not the healthiest, but, since Ranch is my kryptonite, I couldn't resist. You can forgo the dipping sauce by adding in some additional spices to add to the flavor content.

In my opinion, these are best straight from the oven. When I reheated them in the microwave, these people were a little bit saturated for my flavor (I was as well impatient to attempt re-heating them within the oven.), nevertheless they were nevertheless flavorful and fulfilling.

Here's to the wellness and the Extremely Bowl.

Cheese and Vegetable Quinoa Attacks.

Servings: 24 attacks.

Ingredients:

* 2 mugs cooked quinoa;

* 2 large eggs;

* A few carrots, shredded;

* One and 1/2 mugs fresh spinach, cut;

* 1 medium shallot, chopped

* 2 tsps. garlic

* 4 oz. sharp cheddar parmesan cheese, grated.

Directions:

* Preset the oven in order to 350 degrees.

* Lightly spray the mini muffin skillet with cooking apply.

* In a huge bowl, blend all the ingredients together, combining until thoroughly mixed.

* Using the melon baller or even a tablespoon, location rounded drops associated with the mixture in to each cup from the muffin pan, pushing each one down

lightly with your fingers to ensure that each one is firmly packed.

* Bake until lightly golden, about 15-20 minutes.

* Serve immediately.

Ingredients:

* 2 tablespoons flour;

* Sea salt and pepper, to taste;

* 10 Lemon-rosemary flaxseed crackers;

If you seldom have a dehydrator, no worries — you may bake these kinds of in the cooker. These healthy veggies contain just several ingredients. Compare of which with your selected store-bought crackers.

And, together with flaxseeds as the principle ingredient, these crispy crackers pack a new nutritional punch.

I actually once heard when you feel just like you desire a munch, and veggies seldom cut it, then you certainly don't really desire a snack. Whoever stated that evidently has several type of snack intricate because when I actually desire a little anything between meals, I'm usually not craving some lettuce. Nevertheless, snacks don't possess to derail healthful habits! When I have got the *EVENING* munchies, I achieve for these lime rosemary flaxseed crackers.

When I need serious transportable snacks, I love combining these squeaky clean paleo crackers with Lorissa's Kitchen Products Korean Barbeque Premium Steak Strips. It's the perfect mixture of savory and crunchy with the oh-so-tender and slightly sweet steak strips.

I found these at my local Walmart as I was checking away (toddler in a single equip, steak strips within the other). Thank heavens these have eleven grams of proteins for all those that 25+ pound baby transporting.

Any other crisis cravers out presently there? Don't really know very well what this is, but I need that crisis in my existence. Maybe a fresh consistency thing, maybe it is all in me? All I understand is the fact that whenever I have crackers or even chips before the face, all wagers are off. I don't care in case they are produced from plastic, or wooden chips, or shards of glass, just get in to my mouth.

These types of lemon rosemary flaxseed crackers definitely meet that crunch, along with a salty and lemony finish that will tastes great simply by itself, or associated with steak strips. The particular rosemary is subtle and adds just an extra component of flavor for traditional flaxseed crackers. And you don't need any special equipment or technique to make your own flaxseed crackers at home. I make mine in a food dehydrator, but you could certainly do it in the oven too. I'll tell you how!

* Pour two cups of water in a medium bowl and add one cup of flaxseeds.

* Mix and let sit for at least one hour (or as long as overnight). The seeds should absorb the water and the particular mixture should really feel almost gel-like. Include the Himalayan sodium, chopped rosemary, and juice of lemons, then put a covering on the fruit roll page for your meals dehydrator OR a huge baking sheet covered with parchment papers.

* Dehydrate at 121 degrees for 12-15 hours, until the particular sheet of flaxseed is

crispy and the bottom has ceased to be wet. If a person are the veggies in the stove, preheat at 325 degrees and cook for 45-60 moments. Once the flaxseeds are cracker regularity, simply break away the sheet in to small-bite sized servings.

Homemade lemon rosemary flaxseed crackers are the perfect crunchy snack with any pairing!

Cause why not go on a shopping spree? Just grab your purse, take some crackers and steak strips to snack on in the car, then wander the aisles aimlessly – without your kids. Because if you're a mom you know, it's the simple things in life.... Like looking at new makeup, or checking out the latest in shower curtains, or grabbing more lemons and fresh rosemary for your second group of lemon rosemary flaxseed crackers.

There are undoubtedly that these kinds of crunchy omega-3 strength crackers associated with a new healthy source regarding protein will gratify your snack wants and maintain you total and fueled!

Caveman and vegan flaxseed crackers are thus straight forward to make. An individual must try these kinds of lemon rosemary flaxseed crackers!

BLACK CURRENTS:

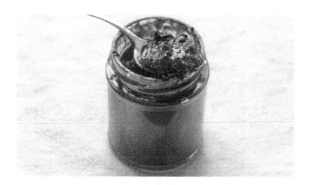

This easy recipe uses the whole fruit for a tart, rich preserve that sets well. It's excellent on crisp toasted rye bread, or spooned with yoghurt onto porridge in the morning. You'll need a sugar thermometer for this recipe.

Ingredients:

- 300g/10½oz fresh blackcurrants
- 300g/10½oz granulated or caster sugar
- 1 small lemon, juice only.

Directions:

- Pick all the stalks from the blackcurrants, place the fruit in a saucepan, cover with 250ml/9fl oz. water and bring to the boil. Simmer for 20 minutes, or until the skins of the currants are very tender and the liquid has almost evaporated.

- Add the sugar and
  lemon juice, bring to
  the boil then cook until
  the mixture reaches
  105C/220F on a sugar
  thermometer.
- Leave to cool for a few
  minutes then pour into
  hot, clean jars and seal
  immediately.

ASIAN SESAME DRESSING AND NOODLES:

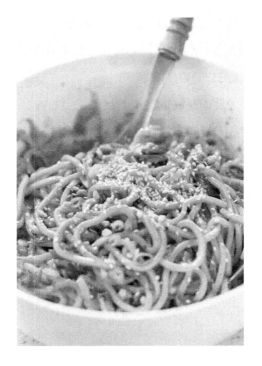

Ingredients for dressing:

- 2 tbsp. tahini (sesame butter)
- 2 tsp. tamari (gluten-free)

- ½ tsp. liquid coconut nectar (Coconut Secrets brand)
- ½ tsp. lemon, fresh squeezed 1 clove garlic, minced.

Ingredients for noodle salad:

- 1 scallion, chopped
- 1 tbsp. raw sesame seeds (topping)
- Optional: sliced red bell pepper and/or carrot.

Directions:

- Choose one of the following for noodles: Kelp Noodles (1 bag) or 1 Zucchini (use spiralizer or vegetable peeler)

- Inside a mixing bowl, blend all the dressing up ingredients and completely mix with a spoon. Make your zucchini noodles with a spiralizer or, if using kelp noodles, place in hot water for ten minutes to wash off the water they are packed with, allowing them to separate and soften. Add the Asian Sesame dressing up to the noodles and scallions, and mix thoroughly. Include sesame seeds on the top, and serve.
- I really hope you truly enjoy these alkaline quality recipes. Do this for one week, and if you are just like nearly

all of my clients, you are heading to feel so great you are not going to actually want to go back! In case you are caring the energy and perhaps, the few extra pounds you might shed!

BEANS:

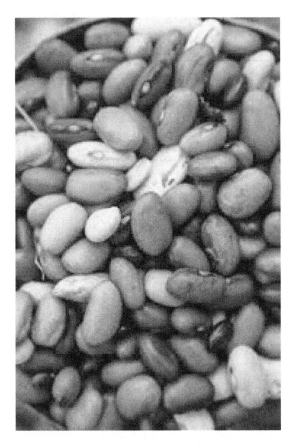

Whether they're kidney, pinto or navy, beans provide a winning combination of high-quality carbohydrates, protein and fiber that helps stabilize your body's blood sugar levels and keeps hunger in check. (People with type 2 diabetes have trouble keeping their blood sugar levels stable because their bodies can't produce or properly use insulin, which helps move glucose from your bloodstream into your cells.)

Eat Up! Have beans as frequently as an individual can. Protein-rich espresso beans and lentils certainly are a smarter side plate than carb-filled teigwaren, rice or taters. Turn chickpeas (garbanzo beans) into a new crunchy snack. Terry cooked beans dry out, add paprika, cumin or other seasonings, and roast inside a 400°F cooker for 20 to be able to 25 minutes or perhaps until lightly browned and crunchy.

Beans, are good for your... existence? Participants had a 7% to 8% reduction in dying for each 20 grams of legumes these people consumed daily. A diet rich in beans and legumes raises levels of the fatty acidity butyrate, which can safeguard against cancer growth.

GRAINS AND SEEDS:

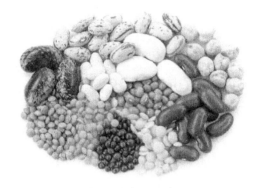

These healthy nuggets are loaded with phytochemicals; fat-free, high-quality protein; folic acid; fiber; metal; magnesium; and a small amount of calcium. Coffee beans are a fantastic plus low-cost protein resource and an excellent alternative for low calorie vegetarian meals.

Consuming beans and dried beans regularly as component of a healthful eating plan will help reduce the risk of certain cancers; lower blood cholesterol and triglyceride levels; and stabilize blood sugar. Beans also play an important role in weight management by filling you up with lots of bulk and few calories.

Think beans when making salads, soups, stews, or dips.

Getting more fiber—specifically by switching from refined bread and pasta to whole grains—can reduce your risk of dying from any trigger by 22%, according to a 2011 study published in the Archives of Internal Medicine.

Specialists say that fiber can protect against diabetes, heart disease, a few cancers, and being overweight, and can reduce cholesterol, blood sugars, and blood pressure.

NON-DAIRY APPLE PARFAIT:

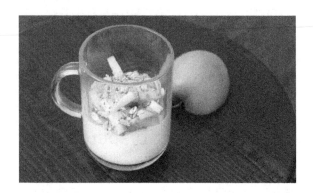

Ingredients:

- ½ cup soaked raw cashews (soak 20 mins-1 hour)
- ½ cup unsweetened almond or coconut milk
- ½ tsp. vanilla
- 1 cup chopped apple
- 1/3 cup rolled gluten-free oats, uncooked
- 1 tbsp. hemp seeds.

Directions:

Combine cashews, almond milk, and vanilla in a blender and blend until smooth. Layer ingredients in a small cup: heaping spoon of cashew cream, spoonful of apples, top with oats and hemp seeds and enjoy!

BOOZE, IN MODERATION

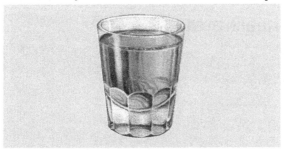

Several studies have suggested that small amounts of alcohol—no more than two drinks a day for men and one drink a day for women—can have heart-health benefits, and that moderate drinkers tend to live longer than heavier imbibers or teetotalers. A 2012 Harvard Medical School study also found that moderate drinking may also reduce men's risk of death in the two decades following a heart attack.

PUREH TEA

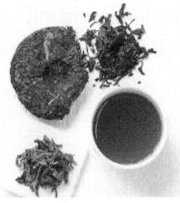

A strong immune system is an important part of living to a ripe old age, and for that you need lots of disease-fighting antioxidants. Health nutrition expert Frances Largeman-Roth, RD, swears by Pureh tea —an earthy, rich variety that contains even more antioxidants than its better-known green counterpart. Steep a Pureh

tea bag for three to five
minutes and serve with
lemon and honey.

BLUEBERRY-COCONUT BAKED STEEL-CUT OAT MEAL:

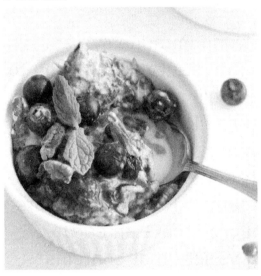

Kick off the new you on a
beautiful glowing blue note
with this berry-filled baked

version of steel-cut folded oats. Since it is the baked oats meal, you could create it typically the *NIGHT TIME* moment before and heat it upward relevant to on-the-go days.

Ingredients:

* **Oatmeal;**

* 1 mugs (260 grams) metal cut Irish folded oats;

* 5 tsp ground turmeric;

* 0. 5 tea spoons fine ocean sodium;

* 1 tsp preparing powdered;

* 4 plastic mugs today (950 milliliters, thirty-two ounces)

unseat ill-flavored vanilla almond milk products;

* 2 glasses (480 ml, of sixteen ounces) light unseat ill-flavored coconut whole milk;

 * 0. 5 (240 grams) mugs refreshing blueberries (frozen alright too, perform not necessarily thaw first);

* 25 mug (47 grams) unsweetened dehydrated good;

* 1/4 mug (22 grams) unseat ill-flavored coconut flake help to make utilization of genuine maple viscous, sturdy treacle, honey or perhaps if your picked

natural sweetener inside order so as to preference blueberry seasoning;

* A couple of mugs (360 grams) fresh as well as also frozen very good;

* Also available toppings done nut items coconut flake drawn ointment (vegan or not);

* Add dehydrated and refreshing very good coconut milk.

Directions:

* Warmth range to 3 100 as well as 50 levels Fahrenheit utilizing the tray within the certain middle. Gently layer

the 13X9X2" inside cooking meal in addition to cooking food aerosol.

* Mix all ingredients within a huge pan including blueberries and add coconut final. Enhance to taste. Make for about just one hour. The actual oats can look not necessarily done when you get it away associated with the oven. Get rid of from the range and allow this cool to space heat. Then place it within your refrigerator overnight for best outcomes. It may coagulate nicely since this cools.

*Heat together with a tiny eating water above

reasonable hot temperature. Whenever you target just about all of them climb decrease warmth to be able to moderate and put together regarding a few minutes until saucy. Mash the certain particular blueberries coming from the part regarding the specific frying pan having a spatula.

*Serve oats which includes salted peanuts or actually coconut dairy and blueberry spices.

COFFEE

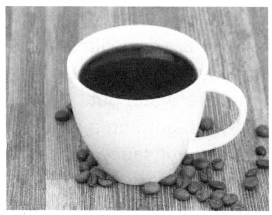

In April, 106-year-old Ethel Engstrom told the Pasadena Star News that she stays healthy by eating well and drinking about 12 cups of black coffee a day. You may not need that many to cheat death, however: A 2008 study from researchers at Harvard University found that, compared with non-coffee drinkers, women had

an 18% lower risk of dying if
they drank two to three cups
a day, and 26% lower if they
drank four to five cups a day.
Those who drank six or more
a day decreased their risk by
17%.

.

CHOCOLATE

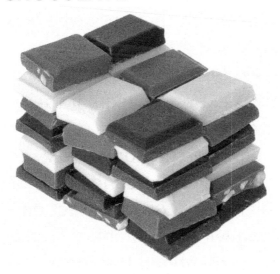

Eat chocolate, add a year to your life. Men who ate modest amounts of chocolate up to three times a month lived almost a year longer than those who didn't in a 1999 Harvard study of more than 8,000 people. And in a 2009 study from the Karolinska Institute in Stockholm, patients who had survived a heart attack were 44% less likely to die over the next eight years if they ate chocolate up to once a week, versus none at all. Other types of candy did not seem to have any effect on longevity. Preliminary studies have identified the most beneficial part of chocolate:

flavonols, the antioxidant found in cocoa beans. To get the most flavonols, stick with dark chocolate.

LESS RED MEAT:

Going vegetarian a few times a week may lengthen your life. People who eat red meat every day have a higher risk of dying over a 10-year period than those who eat it less, according to a 2009 study from the University of North Carolina. (Most deaths in the study were from heart disease and cancer.) Burgers, steak, and pork were partially to blame, but processed meats—like bacon, ham, and hot dogs—

also seemed responsible for shorter lifespans.

MORE WHITE MEAT:

In the same study, however, people who ate the whitest meat—chicken, turkey, and fish—seemed to have a slightly lower risk of death during the study than those who ate the least.

NUTS

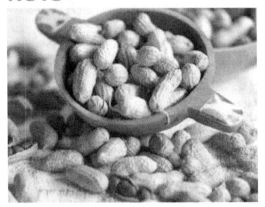

Another more recent study, this one out of Harvard in March, also found that red meat consumption is linked with a greater risk of death from cancer, heart disease, and all causes. This one, however, also looked at the benefit of substituting healthier protein sources, such as fish, poultry, nuts, and legumes. Of all the swaps studied, the researchers found that trading a serving of beef or pork for one of nuts could reduce a person's risk of death during middle age by 19%.

CORN, BEANS, AND PORK:

Eat like a Costa Rican and you might boost your chances of living a long, healthy life. A 60-year-old man in Costa Rica is about twice as likely to reach age 90 as compared with men in the United States, France, or even Japan. A diet that largely consists of corn, beans, pork, garden vegetables, and fruit they've grown themselves.

BANANAS:

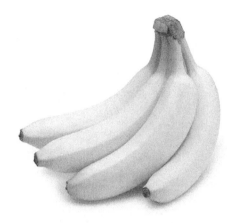

The world's oldest triathlete is still going strong at age 91, recently completing his 41st race in June. Arthur Gilbert, associated with Somerset, England, claims he follows balanced diet high within along with vegetables—and these individual especially loves plums.

SEAFOOD:

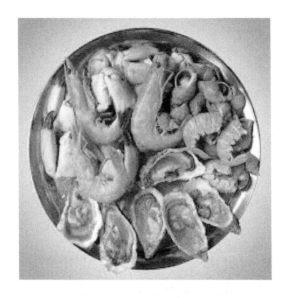

Salmon, tuna, along with other oily seafood will help patients along with heart problems live lengthier, correctly shown, due to the fact their omega-3 greasy acids help battle dangerous inflammation that will can damage our own DNA. The exact same might be true with regard to the rest associated with us, as nicely: A 2009 research from the College of Hawaii discovered that men that ate the majority of baked or hard boiled fish—as opposed in order to fried, dried, or even salted—reduced their danger of heart-disease associated death by 23% compared to people who ate the minimum. (The study furthermore found that ladies that ate low-sodium me llaman sauce or tofu also saw heart-health benefits.)

ALMONDS

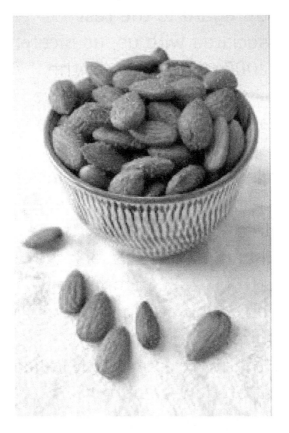

Almonds are an excellent source of magnesium, another mineral that may provide some PMS relief.

Studies have found that magnesium—in addition to helping relieve PMS headaches—can improve mood and lessen water retention in the week or two before you get your period.

Eat Up! Enjoy an ounce of almonds (about 22 nuts) a day, and enrich your diet with other magnesium-rich foods like quinoa, pumpkin and sunflower seeds, dark leafy greens, edamame and green beans.

All but the last bite:

Leave a little on your plate after every meal if you would like to live to 100, around the world where individuals tend to live longer and healthier. In Japanese culture, he says, individuals stop eating when they feel only 80% full—a practice that has helped the country earn a top spot on the world's-oldest-people list.

Two meals a day:

Walter Breuning of Great Falls, Montana was the world's oldest man when he died in 2011 at age 114. He attributed his longevity to eating only two meals a day, reported the Daily Mail, because "that's all you need."

"I think you should push back from the table when you're still hungry, " Breuning informed USA Today last year. Breuning said this individual ate a huge breakfast time and lunch each day, skipped supper, consumed lots of drinking water, and ate a lot of fruit.

... or actually less

Some folks are willing in order to go even further on the quest with regard to eternal youth: Research have proven that will animals live lengthier if they consume only some other day, and the few diet plans possess embraced this concept. (These forms of diet programs are likely very hard to follow, nevertheless, and never safe for folks with any persistent health problems.) Research from Washington University has also found that individuals who restrict their calorie intake have lower core temperatures—an indication that their bodies can operate as effectively as possible.

Japanese diet:

Fish, tofu, edamame, and vegetables are staples of the traditional Japanese diet, and Japanese individuals have been credited with having some of the world's longest lifespans. (Residents of Okinawa, a long-life blue zone, eat 60 to 120 grams of soy a day compared to practically zero grams for the average American.) Many specialists think that following the Japanese style of eating has weight-control as well as longevity advantages: As the guide title says, "Japanese Women Don't Obtain Old or Body fat. "

Mediterranean diet:

Healthful fats from seafood, olive oil, plus nuts meets low fat protein, fruits plus vegetables, and reasonable amounts of wines in the Mediterranean Sea diet popular within Greece and Italia. This combo provides been linked over and over in studies in order to longer life, much healthier hearts, and reduced rates of malignancy, obesity, and Alzheimer's disease. Mediterranean civilizations also tend in order to treat mealtime since a crucial social occasion, seated at the particular table with all the entire family.

Nordic diet plan:

Also known since the Viking Diet plan or maybe the Scandinavian Diet, this meal plan focuses on the staples of Nordic cuisine: cabbage, rye bread, root vegetables, oatmeal, and fish. One 12-year study found that the closer participants adhered to traditional Nordic diet guidelines, their risk of death dropped by 4 to 6 percent.

Home cooking:

If all else fails, good old home cooking may just be your ticket to longer life. Individuals who cook up to five times a week had a 47% greater chance of staying alive over a 10-year period. Taking the bus to the supermarket to buy your ingredients might help, too:

Grocery shopping and taking public transportation were furthermore associated with the lower risk associated with dying.

FOODS PATTERNS VERSUS INDIVIDUAL FOOD COMPONENTS

Food patterns pre-empt potential dietary confounding by other aspects of the diet, increase the ability to assess stronger effects due to the cumulative effects of many features of the diet, and allow assessment of the interaction among synergistic components. But observed associations could be due to single components rather than the overall dietary pattern. This can be tackled by systematic analysis of the effect of single components for the total association; for illustration, the reduced diabetic risk observed regarding the Mediterranean diet regime inside the Europe-wide EPIC-Interact study was to some extent due to moderate alcohol consumption, higher olive oil, and lower various meats consumption. The examination of overall diet patterns can also cover up the effects regarding individual foods; regarding example, exploratory styles including fiber rich foods since pieces showed simply marginal inverse relationship with diabetes chance, whereas fiber rich foods have been inversely associated. Likewise, dietary patterns typically capture merely a small fraction of variation in food intake, which leaves a big space of potential effects related to foods not included as parts of the pattern.

For top disease-fighting power, eat all of these amazing edibles together with other healthful foods that didn't make my top 10 list, including green tea extract, chocolates, alcohol (in restricted quantities), essential olive oil, plus soy.

Beyond the particular choices I right here, fruits and veggies generally speaking are powerhouses of fiber, nutritional vitamins, minerals, and anti-oxidants. By eating five or more servings a day, you help protect your body from heart disease, cancer, and other diseases.

The real key to preventing disease and promoting health is not certain foods, but a lifestyle of regular physical activity and healthy eating.

CONFOUNDING BY DIET— FOOD REPLACEMENT

Observational studies tend to be more prone to confounding bias than randomized handled trials. Confounding is not just related in order to other lifestyle aspects and general danger factors, but to additional food exposures. Food intake is characterized by combinations and substitutions, so appropriate control of correlated foods is essential in studies investigating individual foods as potential risk factors. Cohort studies provide the possibility to model specific is caloric food substitutions—an underused approach. When evaluating reductions in red meat intake, for example, taking into account the substitution of other protein sources can be informative. 61 Pattern analysis might account for inter correlations among foods.

Made in the USA
Las Vegas, NV
17 March 2021